Applied Mixed Model Analysis

This practical book is designed for applied researchers who want to use mixed models with their data. It discusses the basic principles of mixed model analysis, including two-level and three-level structures, and covers continuous outcome variables, dichotomous outcome variables, and categorical and survival outcome variables. Emphasising interpretation of results, the book develops the most important applications of mixed models, such as the study of group differences, longitudinal data analysis, multivariate mixed model analysis, IPD meta-analysis and mixed model predictions. All examples are analysed with STATA, and an extensive overview and comparison of alternative software packages is provided. All datasets used in the book are available for download, so readers can reanalyse the examples to gain a strong understanding of the methods. Although most examples are taken from epidemiological and clinical studies, this book is also highly recommended for researchers working in other fields.

Jos W. R. Twisk specialises in the methodological field of longitudinal data analysis and multilevel/mixed model analysis, about which he has written three textbooks (all published by Cambridge University Press). He has also authored a textbook on applied biostatistics in Dutch. He is the director of the epidemiology masters program of the VU University Medical Center in Amsterdam and head of the Expertise Center for Applied Longitudinal Data Analysis. His main activities include applied methodological research, consulting and teaching courses on mixed model analysis, longitudinal data analysis, multilevel analysis, and applied basic statistics. He has authored or co-authored more than 700 peer-reviewed international papers.

PRACTICAL GUIDES TO BIOSTATISTICS AND EPIDEMIOLOGY

Series advisors

Susan Ellenberg, *University of Pennsylvania School of Medicine*
Robert C. Elston, *Case Western Reserve University School of Medicine*
Brian Everitt, *Institute of Psychiatry, King's College London*
Frank Harrell, *Vanderbilt University School of Medicine, Tennessee*
Jos W. R. Twisk, *University Medical Center, Amsterdam*

This series of short and practical but authoritative books is for biomedical researchers, clinical investigators, public health researchers, epidemiologists, and non-academic and consulting biostatisticians who work with data from biomedical and epidemiological and genetic studies. Some books explore a modern statistical method and its applications, others may focus on a particular disease or condition and the statistical techniques most commonly used in studying it.

The series is for people who use statistics to answer specific research questions. Books will explain the application of techniques, specifically the use of computational tools, and emphasise the interpretation of results, not the underlying mathematical and statistical theory.

Published in the series

Applied Multilevel Analysis Jos W. R. Twisk
Secondary Data Sources for Public Health Sarah Boslaugh
Survival Analysis for Epidemiologic and Medical Research Steve Selvin
Statistical Learning for Biomedical Data James D. Malley, Karen G. Malley and Sinisa Pajevic
Measurement in Medicine Henrica C. W. de Vet, Caroline B. Terwee, Lidwine B. Mokkink and Dirk L. Knol
Preventing and Treating Missing Data in Longitudinal Clinical Trials Craig Mallinckrodt
Genomic Clinical Trials and Predictive Medicine Richard M. Simon

Applied Mixed Model Analysis

A Practical Guide

Jos W.R. Twisk

University Medical Centre Amsterdam

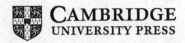

CAMBRIDGE
UNIVERSITY PRESS

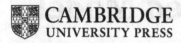

CAMBRIDGE
UNIVERSITY PRESS

Shaftesbury Road, Cambridge CB2 8EA, United Kingdom

One Liberty Plaza, 20th Floor, New York, NY 10006, USA

477 Williamstown Road, Port Melbourne, VIC 3207, Australia

314–321, 3rd Floor, Plot 3, Splendor Forum, Jasola District Centre, New Delhi – 110025, India

103 Penang Road, #05–06/07, Visioncrest Commercial, Singapore 238467

Cambridge University Press is part of Cambridge University Press & Assessment, a department of the University of Cambridge.

We share the University's mission to contribute to society through the pursuit of education, learning and research at the highest international levels of excellence.

www.cambridge.org
Information on this title: www.cambridge.org/9781108727761

DOI: 10.1017/9781108635660

First published 2019

A catalogue record for this publication is available from the British Library

Library of Congress Cataloging-in-Publication data
Names: Twisk, Jos W. R., 1962- author. | Applied multilevel analysis.
Title: Applied mixed model analysis : a practical guide / Jos W.R. Twisk (University Medical Centre Amsterdam).
Description: Second edition. | Cambridge ; New York, NY : Cambridge University Press, 2019. | Series: Practical guides to biostatistics and epidemiology | Continues, in part: Applied multilevel analysis : a practical guide (Cambridge, UK ; New York : Cambridge University Press, 2006). | Includes bibliographical references and index.
Identifiers: LCCN 2018050804 | ISBN 9781108480574 (hardback : alk. paper) | ISBN 9781108727761 (pbk. : alk. paper)
Subjects: LCSH: Medical statistics. | Analysis of variance. | Mathematical statistics.
Classification: LCC QA279 .T95 2019 | DDC 519.5/38–dc23
LC record available at https://lccn.loc.gov/2018050804

ISBN   978-1-108-48057-4   Hardback
ISBN   978-1-108-72776-1   Paperback

To my parents

Contents

Preface

This book is about applied mixed model analysis. The most important word in the title of this book is 'applied'. Before reading this book, it is important to realise that the mathematical background of mixed model analysis will not be discussed in great detail. The emphasis here lies on the application of mixed model analysis. The book addresses questions like: 'In what situations do we need to use mixed model analysis?', 'What kinds of choices do I have to make to perform a proper mixed model analysis?' and 'What do the results of a mixed model analysis actually mean?'

Many books have been written on mixed model analysis, but nearly all of them have been written by statisticians, and therefore they mainly focus on the mathematical background of mixed model analysis. The problem with that approach is that such books are very difficult to understand for non-mathematical researchers. And yet, these non-mathematical researchers are expected to use mixed model analysis to analyse their data. In fact, researchers are primarily interested not in the basic (mostly difficult) mathematical background of the statistical methods, but in finding correct answers to research questions. Furthermore, researchers want to know how to apply a statistical technique and how to interpret the results. Due to their different basic interests and different modes of thinking, communication problems between statisticians and applied researchers are quite common, and they often communicate on different levels. This, in addition to the growing interest in mixed model analysis, motivated the writing of this book. This book is written for non-statistical researchers, and it aims to provide practical guidance on when and how to use mixed model analysis. The purpose of this book is to build a bridge between the different communication levels that exist between statisticians and researchers when addressing the topic of mixed model analysis.

Although the book contains examples that are mostly taken from epidemiological and medical studies, all the methods discussed in this book can be applied to other research fields as well.

1

Introduction

1.1 Introduction

The popularity of applying mixed model analysis has increased rapidly over since around 2005. A very small, non-systematic literature search showed that in 2005, 705 papers were published in which mixed model analysis was applied. In 2010 this number increased to 1292, while in 2016 the number of papers in which mixed model analysis was applied rose to over 2200. Figure 1.1 shows the development from 2005 to 2016 in the number of published papers in which mixed model analysis was applied.

1.2 Background of Mixed Model Analysis

Mixed model analysis was first developed for educational research (Goldstein, 1987, 1992; Goldstein and Cuttance, 1988; Nuttall et al., 1989; Woodhouse and Goldstein, 1989; Plewis, 1991). When analysing the performance of students, the researchers realised that the observations of students in the same class were not independent of each other. Because standard statistical methods assume independent observations, it is not appropriate to use these methods to analyse the performance of students. The structure of such a study can be described as a sort of hierarchy; students are clustered within classes (see Figure 1.2). Because of this hierarchy, mixed model analysis is also known as hierarchical linear modelling.

This situation is known as a two-level data structure, with the first level being the students and the second level being the classes. Because of the different levels, mixed model analysis is also known as multilevel analysis.

Number of publications

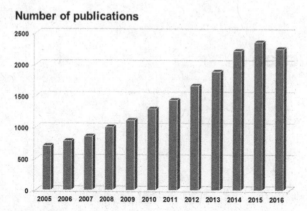

Figure 1.1   Development from 2005 to 2016 in the number of published papers in which mixed model analysis was applied.

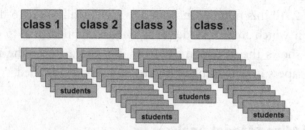

Figure 1.2   Illustration of a two-level hierarchical data structure. Observations of students are clustered within classes.

The general idea of mixed model analysis is that this hierarchy is taken into account in the analysis or, in other words, the analysis takes into account the dependency of the observations. Within the educational setting there can be another (i.e. higher) level of clustering, because not only are the students clustered within classes, but the classes are also clustered within schools (see Figure 1.3). This situation is referred to as a three-level data structure, with the students being level 1, the classes being level 2 and the schools being level 3. Again, the general idea of mixed model analysis in this situation is that it takes into account the dependency of observations, not only within classes, but also within schools.

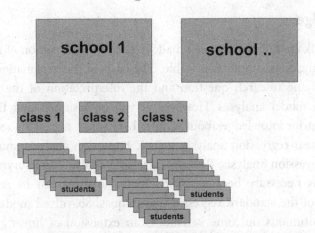

Figure 1.3   Illustration of a three-level hierarchical data structure. Observations of students are clustered within classes and the observations of classes are clustered within schools.

1.3 General Approach

Although there is a considerable amount of basic literature on mixed model analysis, most of it is characterised by a mathematical approach (Bryk and Raudenbush, 1992; Goldstein, 1995, 2003; Kreft and De Leeuw, 1998; Snijders and Bosker, 1999; Little et al., 2000; McCullagh and Searle, 2001; Hox, 2002; Raudenbush and Bryk, 2002; Reise and Duan, 2003; Jiang, 2007, 2016; Demidenko, 2013; Galecki and Burzykowski, 2013; West et al., 2015).

Only a few papers have tried to follow a more practical approach (see, for instance, Korff et al., 1992; Rice and Leyland, 1996; Greenland, 2000a, 2000b; Livert et al., 2001; Diez Roux, 2002; Merlo, 2003; Leyland and Groenewegen, 2003). This book will also follow a more practical approach, which will make it easier to read and more understandable for non-mathematical readers. The emphasis of this book lies on the interpretation of the results of mixed model analysis, on the research questions that can be answered with mixed model analysis, and on the differences between mixed model analysis and the so-called naive approaches that do not take into account the dependency of observations. Therefore, in each chapter, the (mathematically difficult) statistical analyses will be explained by using relatively simple examples, accompanied by computer output.

1.4 Prior Knowledge

In this book an attempt has been made to keep the description of the mixed model analyses as simple as possible. The basis of the explanations will be the underlying research question and the interpretation of the results of the mixed model analyses. However, it will be assumed that the reader has some prior knowledge about standard statistical regression techniques, such as linear regression analysis, logistic regression analysis, multinomial logistic regression analysis, Poisson regression analysis and survival analysis. This is necessary because mixed model analysis can be seen as an extension of the standard regression techniques. So, mixed model analysis with a continuous outcome variable is an extension of linear regression analysis, mixed model analysis with a dichotomous outcome variable is an extension of logistic regression analysis, and so on.

1.5 Example Datasets

All datasets that will be used in the examples will be available from the internet and can be reanalysed by the reader. This will certainly improve understanding of the general theories underlying mixed model analysis.

1.6 Software

All the analyses in the first part of the book are performed with STATA (version 14). In Chapter 13, the use of mixed model analysis in other software packages, such as SPSS, R and SAS, will be discussed. The data used in the examples will be reanalysed with other software and the results will be compared. Both syntax and output will accompany the discussion of the different software packages.

2

Basic Principles of Mixed Model Analysis

2.1 Introduction

The basic principles of mixed model analysis will be explained by using a continuous outcome variable, i.e. they will be explained using a linear mixed model analysis. The most important basic principle to be considered is the fact that linear mixed model analysis can be seen as an extended linear regression analysis. So, to understand the basic principles of mixed model analysis, linear regression analysis must be the starting point.

Suppose that a cohort study is performed to investigate the relationship between physical activity and health. Both are continuous variables and Eq. 2.1 describes the linear regression model. Figure 2.1 illustrates the result of this linear regression analysis.

$$\text{health} = \beta_0 + \beta_1 \text{activity} + \varepsilon \tag{2.1}$$

where 'health' = continuous outcome variable; β_0 = intercept; β_1 = regression coefficient for activity; 'activity' = continuous independent variable and ε = error/residual.

The interpretation of the regression coefficients of this linear regression analysis is very straightforward. The intercept (β_0) is the value of the outcome variable (health) when the independent variable (physical activity) equals zero. The regression coefficient for activity (β_1) reflects the difference in health for subjects who differ one unit in physical activity. Suppose now that the analysis is adjusted for gender. The reason for this adjustment is that males are different from females. Therefore, an adjustment for gender makes sense (Eq. 2.2).

$$\text{health} = \beta_0 + \beta_1 \text{activity} + \beta_2 \text{gender} + \varepsilon \tag{2.2}$$

where β_2 = regression coefficient for gender.

health

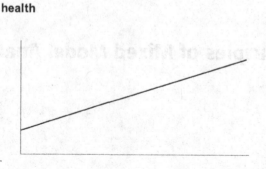

physical activity

Figure 2.1   Illustration of a linear regression analysis of the relationship between physical activity
and health.

health

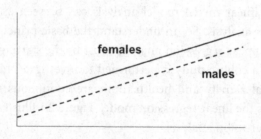

physical activity

Figure 2.2   Illustration of a linear regression analysis of the relationship between physical activity
and health, adjusted for gender.

Suppose that males are coded as 0 and females are coded as 1. The intercept β_0 now reflects the intercept (i.e. the value for health when physical activity equals zero) only for males, while $\beta_0 + \beta_2$ reflects the intercept for females. So, an adjustment for gender actually means that the intercept of the regression line is assumed to be different for males and females (see Figure 2.2).

Suppose another situation in which the study is performed in a city with different neighbourhoods. It is very reasonable to assume that subjects who are living in a particular neighbourhood are more like subjects living in the same neighbourhood than they are like subjects living in other

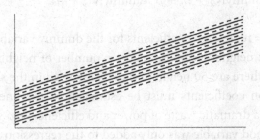

Figure 2.3   Illustration of a linear regression analysis of the relationship between physical activity and health, adjusted for neighbourhood.

neighbourhoods. Subjects can live in a rich neighbourhood or in a poor neighbourhood and the socioeconomic situation of subjects can be related to the outcome of the study (i.e. health). So, because the observations of the outcome variable within a certain neighbourhood are correlated with each other, the linear regression analysis should be adjusted for neighbourhood.

Again, an adjustment for neighbourhood actually means that different intercepts are estimated for each neighbourhood (see Figure 2.3).

When there are many neighbourhoods, the adjustment for neighbourhood raises a problem. When the variable 'neighbourhood' is added to the regression equation as a discrete variable, the regression coefficient for the neighbourhood variable reflects the difference in outcome between neighbourhood number 2 and neighbourhood number 1 but also between neighbourhood number 3 and neighbourhood number 2, etc. In other words, in the analysis with neighbourhood as a discrete variable, a linear relationship between the arbitrary number of the neighbourhood and the outcome variable is assumed. This linear relationship does not make any sense. In fact, the variable neighbourhood is a categorical variable (more specifically a nominal variable), and when an adjustment is made for a categorical variable, it means that dummy variables have to be created. The number of dummy variables depends on the number of neighbourhoods involved in the study (i.e. the number of neighbourhoods minus 1), and for all those dummy variables separate regression coefficients must be estimated (Eq. 2.3).

$$\text{health} = \beta_0 + \beta_1 \text{activity} + \beta_2 \text{dummy}N_1$$
$$+ \beta_3 \text{dummy}N_2 + \dots + \beta_m \text{dummy}N_{m-1} + \varepsilon \qquad (2.3)$$

where β_2 to β_m = regression coefficients for the dummy variables representing the different neighbourhoods, and m = number of neighbourhoods.

Therefore, if there are 50 neighbourhoods involved in the study, 49 additional regression coefficients must be estimated in the linear regression analysis. This is a dramatic waste of power and efficiency, especially because the neighbourhood variable was only added to the regression analysis to be adjusted for. There is no real interest in the different health values for each of the separate neighbourhoods. A much more powerful and efficient way to adjust for neighbourhood is provided by mixed model analysis. The general idea behind a mixed model analysis can be seen as a three-step procedure. In the first step, the intercepts for the different neighbourhoods are estimated. In the second step, a normal distribution is drawn over the different intercepts. In the third step, the variance of that normal distribution is estimated. That variance is then added to the regression model in order to adjust for the neighbourhood. So, instead of estimating 49 regression coefficients to adjust for the neighbourhood, this adjustment is performed by adding only one variance parameter to the model. The estimation of the variance of the intercepts is also referred to as a random intercept. This is why mixed model analysis is also known as random coefficient analysis.

In mixed model terminology it is said that the observations that are made of the subjects are clustered within neighbourhoods. Because the observations of subjects within one neighbourhood are correlated, an adjustment must be made for neighbourhood. In this particular example the data contains a two-level structure: the subject is the lowest level, while the neighbourhood is the highest level (see Figure 2.4).

In general, mixed model analysis is a very efficient way of adjusting for a categorical variable with many categories. Of course, there is some sort of trade-off. This trade-off is the assumption that the distribution of intercepts for the different neighbourhoods is more or less normal, because the variance used in the adjustment is based on the normal distribution. So, when performing a mixed model analysis, it is important to realise that this normality assumption underlies the estimation procedure (see also Section 2.7).

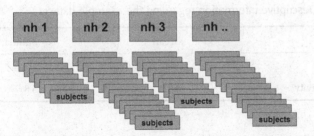

Figure 2.4   Two-level mixed model structure; subjects are clustered within neighbourhoods.

2.2 Example

The example that will be used to explain the basic principles of mixed model analysis is a very simple one: a cross-sectional cohort study investigating the relationship between two continuous variables, physical activity and health. In this study, 684 subjects living in 48 different neighbourhoods are involved. So, in this example, the observations of the subjects are clustered within neighbourhoods. Table 2.1 shows the descriptive information of the data used in this example.

Output 2.1 shows the result of the standard linear regression analysis without adjusting for the neighbourhood. This kind of analysis is also referred to as a naive regression analysis because it ignores the possible clustering of data, meaning it ignores the fact that the observations of subjects within the same neighbourhood can be correlated.

The same result can also be obtained from a so-called naive mixed model analysis: a mixed model analysis without adjusting for the neighbourhood. Output 2.2 shows the result of this analysis.

The first line of Output 2.2 shows that a mixed effects maximum-likelihood (ML) regression is performed. The first part of the right-hand column refers to the number of observations (684). In the last line of the left-hand column, the log likelihood is given. The log likelihood value is a result of the maximum-likelihood estimation procedure. The value itself is not informative but can be used in the likelihood ratio test. The first part of the output also gives the result of a statistical test. This test is a Chi-square test with one degree of freedom. The Chi-square value is 241.24 with a corresponding p-value <0.001. This is the result of a statistical test for all the variables in the model. In this analysis, the only variable in the model is

Table 2.1 Descriptive information regarding the example dataset

	Mean	Standard deviation
Health	30.3	6.7
Physical activity	50.2	5.8

Output 2.1 Result of a standard linear regression analysis of the relationship between physical activity and health

```
    Source |       SS           df       MS              Number of obs   =      684
-------------+----------------------------------          F(1, 682)       =   240.54
       Model |  8020.05734         1  8020.05734          Prob > F        =   0.0000
    Residual |  22739.5728       682  33.3424821          R-squared       =   0.2607
-------------+----------------------------------          Adj R-squared   =   0.2596
       Total |  30759.6301       683  45.0360617          Root MSE        =   5.7743


      health |      Coef.   Std. Err.      t    P>|t|     [95% Conf. Interval]
-------------+----------------------------------------------------------------
    activity |   .5933817     .03826    15.51   0.000     .5182603    .6685032
       _cons |   .5743945    1.93192     0.30   0.766    -3.21883    4.367619
```

Output 2.2 Result of a naive linear mixed model analysis of the relationship between physical activity and health, i.e. without an adjustment for neighbourhood

```
Mixed-effects ML regression                     Number of obs    =       684

                                                Wald chi2(1)     =    241.24
Log likelihood = -2168.8891                     Prob > chi2      =    0.0000


      health |      Coef.   Std. Err.      z    P>|z|     [95% Conf. Interval]
-------------+----------------------------------------------------------------
    activity |   .5933817    .038204    15.53   0.000     .5185033    .6682602
       _cons |   .5743945   1.929093     0.30   0.766    -3.206559    4.355348


Random-effects Parameters  |   Estimate   Std. Err.     [95% Conf. Interval]
---------------------------+--------------------------------------------------
              var(Residual) |   33.24499   1.797683      29.90188    36.96187
```

activity. It should be noted that in general this statistical test does not provide interesting information.

The second part of the output shows the regression coefficients. This part is also referred to as the fixed part of the regression model. Besides the regression coefficient, the standard error, the z-value (which is calculated as the regression coefficient divided by the standard error), the corresponding p-value and the 95% confidence interval (CI) are given. The 95% CI is calculated as the regression coefficient ±1.96 times the standard error. The regression coefficient for activity (0.5933817) reflects the difference in health when there is one unit difference in physical activity. The intercept (0.5743945) reflects the value of health when physical activity equals 0. It should be noted that the value of the intercept in this example is not informative, because there is no physical activity equals 0 in the example dataset. The z-value for the test whether the regression coefficient for activity equals 0 is 15.53. The squared value of this number gives 241.50, which is exactly the same as the value given in the first part of the output that was used as a test statistic for all variables in the model. It should be noted that the Chi-square distribution with one degree of freedom is equal to the standard normal distribution squared. So, the z-test for the variable activity gives exactly the same p-value as the Chi-square test for all variables in the model.

The last part of the output shows the so-called random part of the regression model. Because a naive mixed model analysis was performed, the random part of the regression model only contains the residual variance, which is also known as the error variance or the unexplained variance.

In the second step of the example analysis, an adjustment is made for neighbourhood; in other words, a random intercept on the neighbourhood level is added to the model. As mentioned before, this is done by estimating the variance of the intercepts for the different neighbourhoods (based on a normal distribution). Output 2.3 shows the result of this analysis.

In the first part of Output 2.3 it can be seen that the group variable neighbourhood is added to the model and that there are 48 neighbourhoods. The right-hand column also shows the average number of subjects in a particular neighbourhood (14.3) and the minimum and maximum number of subjects (4 and 49 subjects, respectively).

The fixed part of the regression model provides the same information as before, although the numbers are slightly different, because in the analysis reported in Output 2.3 an adjustment for neighbourhood has been made. That adjustment can be found in the random part of the regression model, which now contains not only the residual variance but also the random intercept variance (4.018727). This number reflects the variance in

Output 2.3 Result of a linear mixed model analysis of the relationship between physical activity and health, with a random intercept on neighbourhood level

```
Mixed-effects ML regression                    Number of obs    =        684
Group variable: neighbourhood                  Number of groups =         48

                                               Obs per group:
                                                            min =          4
                                                            avg =       14.3
                                                            max =         49

                                               Wald chi2(1)     =     241.50
Log likelihood = -2153.4088                    Prob > chi2      =     0.0000

------------------------------------------------------------------------------
      health |     Coef.   Std. Err.      z    P>|z|     [95% Conf. Interval]
-------------+----------------------------------------------------------------
    activity |   .5896818    .037945    15.54   0.000     .515311    .6640527
       _cons |   .7898844   1.941018     0.41   0.684    -3.01444    4.594209
------------------------------------------------------------------------------


------------------------------------------------------------------------------
  Random-effects Parameters  |   Estimate   Std. Err.     [95% Conf. Interval]
-----------------------------+------------------------------------------------
neighbourhood: Identity      |
                 var(_cons)  |   4.018727   1.359694     2.070587    7.799802
-----------------------------+------------------------------------------------
               var(Residual) |   29.57958   1.661547     26.49587    33.02218
------------------------------------------------------------------------------
LR test vs. linear model: chibar2(01) = 30.96       Prob >= chibar2 = 0.0000
```

intercepts for the different neighbourhoods around the intercept value given in the fixed part of the model (0.7898844). The variance is estimated from a normal distribution around the intercepts of all the different neighbourhoods (see Section 2.1).

The question then arises whether or not it is necessary to adjust for neighbourhood, or in other words, whether or not a random intercept should be added to the model. This question can be answered by performing the likelihood ratio test. The likelihood ratio test compares the -2 log likelihood of the model with a random intercept and the -2 log likelihood of the model without a random intercept. The difference between the -2 log likelihoods of the two models follows a Chi-square distribution. The number of degrees of freedom for this Chi-square distribution is equal to the difference in the number of parameters estimated in the two models. In the present example the difference between the two -2 log likelihoods equals:

$$(-2 \times -2168.8891) - (-2 \times -2153.4088) = 4337.7782 - 4306.8176 = 30.96$$

which follows a Chi-square distribution with one degree of freedom. There is one degree of freedom because, compared to the naive analysis, in the second analysis only the variance of the intercepts is additionally estimated, which is only one parameter. Because the critical value for a Chi-square distribution with one degree of freedom is 3.84, the difference of 30.96 is highly significant. It is argued that when variance parameters are added to the model, the difference between the two $-2 \log$ likelihoods should be tested one sided. Because a variance can only be positive the difference between the $-2 \log$ likelihoods can only be in one direction (Goldstein, 1995, 2003; Lin, 1997). It is rather strange that for the likelihood ratio test in mixed model analysis one-sided p-values are used, while for likelihood ratio tests in standard logistic or Cox-regression analysis, for instance, two-sided p-values are used. In these standard situations basically the same phenomenon occurs, because adding variables to models can only lead to a $-2 \log$ likelihood change in one direction. Although in practice it is not really a big deal whether one-sided or two-sided p-values are used, it is important to realise that this contradiction exists in the literature. In the remaining part of this book two-sided p-values will be used for the likelihood ratio tests.

The result of the likelihood ratio test to compare the model with a random intercept and the model without a random intercept (i.e. a standard linear regression analysis) can also be found in the last line of the output.

The most interesting information in the output is still the fixed part of the regression model, which shows the regression coefficient for activity. Adjusted for neighbourhood, the regression coefficient for activity is 0.586818. So, a difference of one unit in activity between subjects is associated with a difference of 0.59 units in the continuous health outcome. When the z-test is performed for this regression coefficient, it is obvious that this relationship is highly significant. The 95% CI around the regression coefficient of 0.59 ranges from 0.52 to 0.66.

2.3 Intraclass Correlation Coefficient

Based on the random intercept variance and the residual variance, the so-called intraclass correlation coefficient (ICC) can be calculated. This ICC is an indication of the average correlation of the observations of subjects living in the same neighbourhood. The ICC is defined as the variance between neighbourhoods divided by the total variance, where the total variance is defined as the summation of the variance between neighbourhoods and the variance within neighbourhoods. The variance within neighbourhoods is equal to the residual variance. It seems to be counterintuitive that a correlation coefficient is calculated from variances. Therefore, Figure 2.5 illustrates this phenomenon. Figure 2.5a shows the distribution of a particular outcome variable, and in Figure 2.5b and c the outcome variable is divided into three groups (for instance three different neighbourhoods). In Figure 2.5b, the ICC is low, because the variance within groups is high and the variance between groups is low. Because in Figure 2.5c the groups are more spread out, the between-group variance increases and the within-group variance decreases. As a consequence, the ICC is high. In fact, Figure 2.5c shows the most extreme situation given the data, i.e. there is maximal between-group variance and minimal within-group variance, leading to the highest possible ICC, given the variance in the data. Thus, in fact, variance and correlation are related to each other one to one.

Going back to the results of the example given in Output 2.3, the ICC can be calculated by dividing the between-neighbourhood variance (4.018727) by the total variance, which is calculated by summation of the between-neighbourhood variance and the within-neighbourhood variance (4.018727 + 29.57958). So, in this example the ICC is 4.02/33.6 = 0.12. It should be noted that this ICC is not the pure ICC present in the data, because both variances are calculated from a model which includes the independent variable physical activity. Physical activity is related to the outcome health, so it reduces the remaining residual variance considerably. Besides that, it is possible that physical activity also explains some of the differences between the neighbourhoods, so the between-neighbourhood variance can also be influenced by physical activity. Therefore, it is better to calculate the pure ICC, which can be done with a so-called intercept-only model (i.e. a model with an intercept but without any independent variables). This intercept-only model has to include an adjustment for the neighbourhood, meaning it has to include a random intercept. Output 2.4 shows the result of this analysis.

Output 2.4 shows that both the random intercept variance and the residual variance are higher compared to the model with physical activity (Output 2.3). From the numbers given in Output 2.4 the pure ICC can be

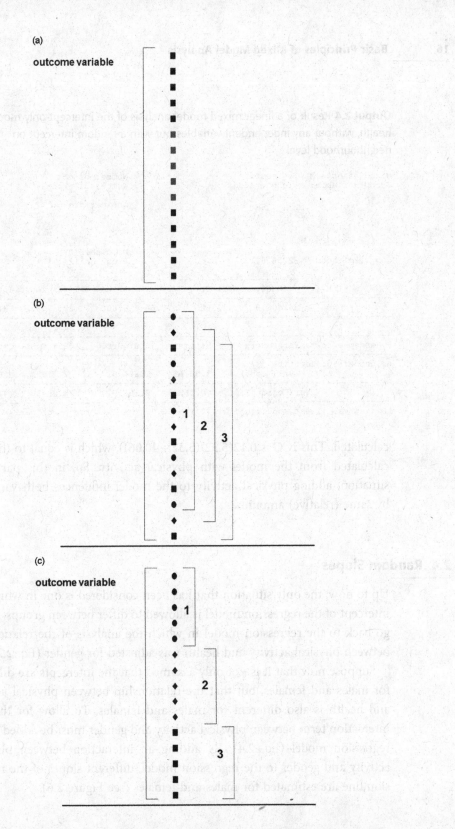

Figure 2.5   Illustration of the intraclass correlation coefficient (ICC). The higher the variance within the groups, the lower the ICC.

Output 2.4 Result of a linear mixed model analysis of the intercept-only model for health, without any independent variables but with a random intercept on neighbourhood level

```
Mixed-effects ML regression                    Number of obs    =        684
Group variable: neighbourhood                  Number of groups =         48

                                               Obs per group:
                                                            min =          4
                                                            avg =       14.3
                                                            max =         49

                                               Wald chi2(0)     =          .
Log likelihood = -2256.8213                    Prob > chi2      =          .

------------------------------------------------------------------------------
      health |      Coef.   Std. Err.      z    P>|z|     [95% Conf. Interval]
-------------+----------------------------------------------------------------
       _cons |   30.40879   .4243625    71.66   0.000     29.57705    31.24052
------------------------------------------------------------------------------


------------------------------------------------------------------------------
  Random-effects Parameters  |   Estimate   Std. Err.     [95% Conf. Interval]
-----------------------------+------------------------------------------------
neighbourh~d: Identity       |
                 var(_cons)  |   5.321694   1.824091      2.71824    10.41866
-----------------------------+------------------------------------------------
               var(Residual) |   40.06234   2.251191      35.88438   44.72674
------------------------------------------------------------------------------
LR test vs. linear model: chibar2(01) = 30.77        Prob >= chibar2 = 0.0000
```

calculated. This ICC is 0.12(5.32/(5.32 + 40.06)), which is equal to the ICC calculated from the model with physical activity. So, in this particular situation, adding physical activity to the model influences both variances by same (relative) amount.

2.4 Random Slopes

Up to now, the only situation that has been considered is one in which the intercept of the regression model is allowed to differ between groups. Let us go back to the regression model in which the analysis of the relationship between physical activity and health was adjusted for gender (Eq. 2.2).

Suppose now that it is not only assumed that the intercepts are different for males and females, but that the relationship between physical activity and health is also different for males and females. To allow for that, an interaction term between physical activity and gender must be added to the regression model (Eq. 2.4). By adding an interaction between physical activity and gender to the regression model, different slopes of the regression line are estimated for males and females (see Figure 2.6).

health

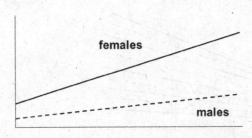

physical activity

Figure 2.6   Illustration of a linear regression analysis of the relationship between physical activity and health, with an interaction between physical activity and gender.

$$\text{health} = \beta_0 + \beta_1 \text{activity} + \beta_2 \text{gender} + \beta_3 (\text{activity} \times \text{gender}) + \varepsilon \qquad (2.4)$$

where β_3 = regression coefficient for the interaction between physical activity and gender.

When the possible effect modifier (i.e. gender) is a dichotomous variable, just one interaction term has to be added to the regression model. However, when it is not the interaction with gender that is of interest, but for instance the interaction with neighbourhood, the same problems that were described for the adjustment for neighbourhood arise. When the observations are clustered within neighbourhoods, it may be reasonable to assume that the relationship between physical activity and health is different for different neighbourhoods. In other words, in this situation different slopes of the regression line have to be estimated for each neighbourhood (see Figure 2.7).

In a standard linear regression analysis this can be done by adding interaction terms between physical activity and the dummy variables representing the different neighbourhoods to the regression model (Eq. 2.5).

$$\begin{aligned}\text{health} = \ &\beta_0 + \beta_1 \text{activity} + \beta_2 \text{dummyN}_1 + \cdots + \beta_m \text{dummyN}_{m-1} \\ &+ \beta_{m+1}(\text{activity} \times \text{dummyN}_2) + \cdots \\ &+ \beta_{2m-1}(\text{activity} \times \text{dummyN}_{m-1}) + \varepsilon\end{aligned} \qquad (2.5)$$

where β_{m+1} to β_{2m-1} = regression coefficients for the interactions between physical activity and the dummy variables representing the different neighbourhoods, and m = number of neighbourhoods.

health

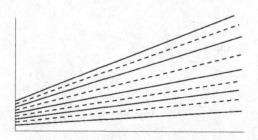

physical activity

Figure 2.7   Illustration of a linear regression analysis of the relationship between physical activity and health, with an interaction between physical activity and neighbourhood.

In this example with 48 neighbourhoods, 47 interaction terms have to be added to the regression model. Estimating 47 regression coefficients that are not of major interest will, again, lead to a loss of power and efficiency. Comparable to what has been described for the different intercepts, the interest is in the overall relationship between physical activity and health. To cope with this, mixed model analysis provides a very elegant solution, and it does so for this situation as well. As for the different intercepts, a three-step procedure can be applied. First, different regression coefficients for the relationship between physical activity and health are estimated for the different neighbourhoods. Then, a normal distribution is drawn over the different regression coefficients. Finally, the variance of the normal distribution is estimated. Now only one variance parameter reflects the difference in the relationship between physical activity and health for the different neighbourhoods. So, in addition to a random intercept, a random slope can also be considered. Again, it should be noted that the estimation of the variance of the slopes is based on a normal distribution.

2.5 Example

Let us go back to the example dataset that was described in Section 2.2. Output 2.5 shows the output of the mixed model analysis on the example dataset in which not only a random intercept is added to the model, but also a random slope for physical activity.

Output 2.5 Result of a linear mixed model analysis of the relationship between physical activity and health, with both a random intercept and a random slope for activity at neighbourhood level

```
Mixed-effects ML regression                Number of obs     =        684
Group variable: neighbourhood              Number of groups  =         48

                                           Obs per group:
                                                        min =          4
                                                        avg =       14.3
                                                        max =         49

                                           Wald chi2(1)      =     241.50
Log likelihood = -2153.4088                Prob > chi2       =     0.0000

-------------------------------------------------------------------------
      health |     Coef.   Std. Err.      z    P>|z|    [95% Conf. Interval]
-------------+-----------------------------------------------------------
    activity |   .5896818    .037945   15.54   0.000    .515311    .6640527
       _cons |   .7898843   1.941018    0.41   0.684   -3.01444   4.594209
-------------------------------------------------------------------------


-------------------------------------------------------------------------
  Random-effects Parameters  |   Estimate   Std. Err.    [95% Conf. Interval]
-----------------------------+-------------------------------------------
neighbourhood: Independent   |
                var(activity)|   5.02e-18    3.11e-17    2.63e-23    9.57e-13
                var(_cons)   |   4.01872    1.359693    2.070582    7.799793
-----------------------------+-------------------------------------------
                var(Residual)|  29.57958    1.661548    26.49587   33.02218
-------------------------------------------------------------------------
LR test vs. linear model: chi2(2) = 30.96            Prob > chi2 = 0.0000
```

The first two parts of Output 2.5 (i.e. the general information and the fixed part of the regression model) look exactly the same as the output of the mixed model analysis with only a random intercept on neighbourhood level (see Output 2.3). The difference between the two outputs is found in the random part of the regression model. It can be seen that on the neighbourhood level the 'var(activity)' is added. This is the random slope variance for activity, i.e. the variance over the regression coefficients for physical activity for the different neighbourhoods. This variance is a very small number, but that does not necessarily mean that the random slope for physical activity is not important. To evaluate the importance of the random slope for activity, a likelihood ratio test must be performed.

The $-2 \log$ likelihood of the model with both a random intercept and a random slope for physical activity is $-2 \times -2153.4088 = 4306.8$. Compared to the $-2 \log$ likelihood of the model with only a random intercept (4306.8), adding a random slope to the model did not lead to a significant improvement of the model. Therefore, it is not necessary to add a random slope for physical activity to the model. From Output 2.5 it can

Output 2.6 Result of a linear mixed model analysis of the relationship between physical activity and health, with both a random intercept and a random slope for activity at neighbourhood level, without assuming that the random coefficients are independent

```
Mixed-effects ML regression                  Number of obs    =        684
Group variable: neighbourhood                Number of groups =         48

                                             Obs per group:
                                                          min =          4
                                                          avg =       14.3
                                                          max =         49

                                             Wald chi2(1)     =     143.47
Log likelihood = -2142.4879                  Prob > chi2      =     0.0000

------------------------------------------------------------------------------
      health |    Coef.    Std. Err.      z    P>|z|    [95% Conf. Interval]
-------------+----------------------------------------------------------------
    activity |  .5901676   .0492719    11.98   0.000    .4935964    .6867389
       _cons |  .7684219   2.713255     0.28   0.777   -4.54946    6.086304
------------------------------------------------------------------------------


------------------------------------------------------------------------------
  Random-effects Parameters  |   Estimate   Std. Err.    [95% Conf. Interval]
-----------------------------+------------------------------------------------
neighbourhood: Unstructured  |
               var(activity) |   .0455139   .0233604      .016644      .12446
                 var(_cons)  |   166.4141   71.09505     72.03468    384.4488
          cov(activity,_cons)|  -2.750856   1.283175    -5.265833   -.2358778
-----------------------------+------------------------------------------------
               var(Residual) |   27.98557   1.61553     24.99175    31.33803
------------------------------------------------------------------------------
LR test vs. linear model: chi2(3) = 52.80           Prob > chi2 = 0.0000
```

also be seen that the random slope for activity and the random intercept are assumed to be independent. It is questionable whether it makes sense to assume the two random components are independent. Because they belong to the same neighbourhood, it is expected that the intercept and slope for a particular neighbourhood are related to each other. Therefore, it makes more sense to model this dependency together with the random slope for physical activity. Output 2.6 shows the results of a mixed model analysis in which the random intercept and the random slope for activity are not assumed to be independent.

From the random part of the regression model in Output 2.6 it can be seen that besides the random intercept and the random slope for activity, the covariance between the random intercept and random slope for activity '(cov(activity,_cons))' is modelled as well. It can also be seen that the random slope variance for activity is much higher than the random slope variance given in Output 2.5 as well as that the random intercept variance has increased enormously. The next step is to compare the two models with each other by using the likelihood ratio test. It is common to compare the model presented in Output 2.6 (i.e. the model with a random slope and the covariance between random intercept and slope) with the model with only a random intercept (Output 2.3). The -2 log likelihood of the model with a random intercept, a random slope for activity and the covariance between the random intercept and random slope is $-2 \times -2142.4879 = 4285$. When this value is compared with the -2 log likelihood of the model with only a random intercept (i.e. 4306.8) it can be seen that there is an improvement of more than 21 points. This value has to be evaluated on a Chi-square distribution of two degrees of freedom, because besides the random slope for activity, the covariance between the random intercept and the random slope for activity also was added to the model. The critical value of the Chi-square distribution with two degrees of freedom is 5.99, so the model with a random intercept, a random slope for activity and the covariance between the random intercept and the random slope, is significantly better than the model with only a random intercept. It should be noted that the model assuming independence between a random intercept and a random slope on the same level does not makes much sense, so it is advised not to assume independence between the two random components on the same level, but to always model the dependency together with the new random component.

The covariance between the random intercept and the random slope is also known as the correlation between the random intercept and the random slope or the interaction between the random intercept and the random slope. For the interpretation of this covariance, the sign is probably the most important. In the example the covariance has a negative sign, which indicates an inverse relationship between the random intercept and the random slope for activity. In other words, for neighbourhoods with a relatively high intercept, a relatively low slope is observed (see Figure 2.8). On the other hand, a positive sign of the covariance between a random intercept and a random slope indicates that the group with a relatively high intercept also has a relatively high slope.

Looking at Output 2.6 and Output 2.3, it was already mentioned that the random intercept variance in the model with only a random intercept is much lower than the random intercept variance in the model with a random intercept, a random slope and the covariance between the random intercept and the random slope (i.e. 4.0 versus 166.4). The high value of the

health

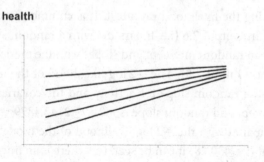

physical activity

Figure 2.8   Illustration of a situation with a negative covariance between a random intercept and a random slope; neighbourhoods with a relatively high intercept have a relatively low slope.

random intercept variance in the model with a random intercept, a random slope and the covariance between a random slope and a random intercept has to do with the fact that the intercept in this example does not have a real interpretation. As mentioned before, the value of the intercept indicates the value of the outcome 'variable health' when the independent variable 'physical activity' equals zero. In the example dataset, the physical activity score ranges between 29 and 61. Therefore, the intercept reflects a value which is far from the observed values. In a situation with only a random intercept this does not influence the variance between the intercepts, because the difference between the regression lines is equal at each value for physical activity (see Figure 2.9a). However, when the slopes of the regression lines differ, this can have a major influence on the variance of the intercepts when the value of the intercept is non-informative (see Figure 2.9b).

A possible way in which to make the intercept more interpretable is to use the centred value of the independent variable in the analysis. This can be done by subtracting the average activity score from all individual observations. Because the result of this subtraction is that the average activity score in the dataset will be zero, the intercept can be interpreted as the outcome variable health for the average physical activity score. Output 2.7 shows the result of a mixed model analysis with a random intercept, a random slope for physical activity and the covariance between the random intercept and slope, when physical activity is centred.

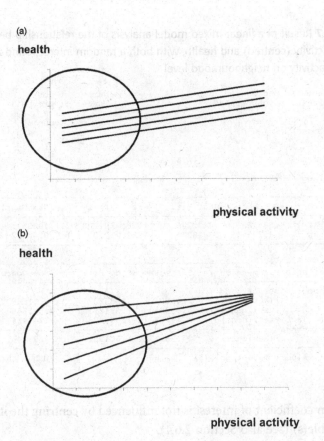

Figure 2.9   (a) Illustration of a mixed model analysis with only a random intercept. Differences between the regression lines are the same for all values of the independent variable. (b) Illustration of a mixed model analysis with both a random intercept and a random slope. Differences between the regression lines are different for different values of the independent variable.

From Output 2.7 it can be seen that the regression coefficient (and random variance) for activity is, of course, exactly the same as before, but the magnitude of the intercept and the random intercept variance have changed considerably. It can further be seen that the random intercept variance has more or less the same value as in the analysis with only a random intercept. To make the intercept and the random intercept variance better interpretable, it is often argued that for all mixed model analyses, the independent variables should be centred. It should be noted that the

Output 2.7 Result of a linear mixed model analysis of the relationship between physical activity (centred) and health, with both a random intercept and a random slope for activity on neighbourhood level

```
Mixed-effects ML regression                    Number of obs     =        684
Group variable: neighbourhood                  Number of groups  =         48

                                               Obs per group:
                                                             min =          4
                                                             avg =       14.3
                                                             max =         49

                                               Wald chi2(1)      =     143.45
Log likelihood = -2142.4879                    Prob > chi2       =     0.0000

------------------------------------------------------------------------------
     health |      Coef.   Std. Err.      z    P>|z|     [95% Conf. Interval]
------------+-----------------------------------------------------------------
activity_c~t |    .5901689   .0492746    11.98   0.000    .4935925    .6867453
      _cons |   30.37344    .3928229    77.32   0.000   29.60352    31.14336
------------------------------------------------------------------------------


------------------------------------------------------------------------------
  Random-effects Parameters   |   Estimate   Std. Err.    [95% Conf. Interval]
------------------------------+-----------------------------------------------
neighbourhood: Unstructured   |
               var(activi~t)  |   .0455241   .0233207      .01668    .1242473
               var(_cons)     |   4.958736   1.551291    2.685846    9.155051
         cov(activi~t,_cons)  |  -.467691    .1567888   -.7749914   -.1603905
------------------------------+-----------------------------------------------
               var(Residual)  |  27.98527   1.614951    24.99246    31.33646
------------------------------------------------------------------------------
LR test vs. linear model: chi2(3) = 52.80             Prob > chi2 = 0.0000
```

regression coefficient of interest is not influenced by centring the independent variable(s) (see also Section 2.6.1).

2.6 Mixed Model Analysis with More than Two Levels

Up to now, only a relatively simple situation has been considered in which the individual observations were clustered within neighbourhoods. It is, however, also possible that the different neighbourhoods are clustered within, for instance, regions (see Figure 2.10).

It is not surprising that this clustering within a higher level can be treated in the same way as has been described for the clustering of the individual observations within neighbourhoods. So, for the different regions, a random intercept (i.e. the variance of the intercepts for the different regions) and a random slope for activity (i.e. the variance of the regression coefficients for activity for the different regions) can also be estimated. It should be realised that, in general, the model building procedure starts by adding random

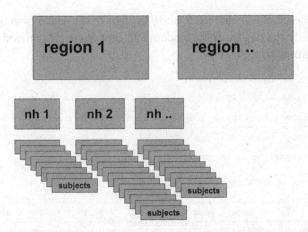

Figure 2.10 Three-level mixed model structure; subjects are clustered within neighbourhoods and neighbourhoods are clustered within regions.

intercepts on the different levels to the model step by step and, after that, possible random slopes are considered.

2.6.1 Example

Output 2.8 shows the result of a mixed model analysis in which a random intercept is assumed for neighbourhood as well as for region.

From the first part of Output 2.8 it can be seen that the outcome variable is measured on three levels, subjects, neighbourhoods and regions, and that there are 12 regions. The model with a random intercept on the region level and a random intercept on the neighbourhood level can be seen as an extension of the model with only a random intercept on neighbourhood level, the result of which was shown in Output 2.3. The difference between the two can be found in the random part of the regression model. Here, we see the random intercept variance on region level (2.947866) and the random intercept variance on neighbourhood level (1.128718). The necessity of the additional random intercept on region level can be evaluated with the likelihood ratio test. Therefore, the $-2\log$ likelihood of the model with only a random intercept on neighbourhood level ($-2 \times -2153.4088 = 4306.8176$) has to be compared to the $-2\log$ likelihood of the model with both a random intercept on neighbourhood and region level ($-2 \times -2146.8629 = 4293.7258$). This difference is 13.09 and evaluated on a Chi-square distribution

Output 2.8 Result of a linear mixed model analysis of the relationship between physical activity and health, with a random intercept on neighbourhood level and a random intercept on region level

```
Mixed-effects ML regression                      Number of obs    =        684

---------------------------------------------------------------------------
                |  No. of          Observations per Group
 Group Variable |  Groups    Minimum     Average     Maximum
----------------+----------------------------------------------------------
         region |     12        22         57.0          84
   neighbourh~d |     48         4         14.3          49
---------------------------------------------------------------------------

                                             Wald chi2(1)     =     236.16
Log likelihood = -2146.8629                  Prob > chi2      =     0.0000

---------------------------------------------------------------------------
       health |    Coef.   Std. Err.      z    P>|z|     [95% Conf. Interval]
--------------+------------------------------------------------------------
     activity |  .579524   .0377111    15.37   0.000     .5056115    .6534364
        _cons |   1.4913   1.980434     0.75   0.451    -2.390279    5.372879
---------------------------------------------------------------------------


---------------------------------------------------------------------------
  Random-effects Parameters  |  Estimate   Std. Err.     [95% Conf. Interval]
-----------------------------+---------------------------------------------
region: Identity             |
                var(_cons)   |  2.947866   1.569788      1.038075    8.371184
-----------------------------+---------------------------------------------
neighbourh~d: Identity       |
                var(_cons)   |  1.128718   .7955629      .2835481    4.493081
-----------------------------+---------------------------------------------
              var(Residual)  |  29.50382   1.65266       26.43615    32.92748
---------------------------------------------------------------------------
LR test vs. linear model: chi2(2) = 44.05          Prob > chi2 = 0.0000
```

with one degree of freedom. This difference is highly statistically significant, so a random intercept on region level is necessary. Looking at the two variances provided in Output 2.8 it can be seen that most of the between-neighbourhood variance shown in Output 2.3 (the linear mixed model analysis with only a random intercept on neighbourhood level) is actually the variance between regions. Only a relatively small part of the variance is still related to the neighbourhoods. The latter now reflects the difference in health between neighbourhoods within regions.

The next step in the modelling procedure is to add a random slope for activity on neighbourhood level to the model. Output 2.9 shows the result of this analysis.

From the random part of the regression model in Output 2.9 it can be seen that a random slope for activity on the neighbourhood level is added to the model. It can also be seen that the covariance between the random intercept and the random slope for activity on the neighbourhood level is

Output 2.9 Result of a linear mixed model analysis of the relationship between physical activity and health, with both a random intercept and a random slope for activity on neighbourhood level and with a random intercept on region level

```
Mixed-effects ML regression                    Number of obs     =         684

-----------------------------------------------------------------------------
                    |    No. of      Observations per Group
 Group Variable |    Groups   Minimum    Average    Maximum
--------------------+--------------------------------------------------------
         region |        12        22       57.0         84
    neighbourh~d |        48         4       14.3         49
-----------------------------------------------------------------------------
                                               Wald chi2(1)      =      144.82
Log likelihood = -2141.5435                    Prob > chi2       =      0.0000

-----------------------------------------------------------------------------
       health |      Coef.   Std. Err.      z    P>|z|     [95% Conf. Interval]
--------------+--------------------------------------------------------------
     activity |   .5824125   .0483976    12.03   0.000      .487555      .67727
        _cons |   1.272692   2.624986     0.48   0.628    -3.872185    6.417569
-----------------------------------------------------------------------------


-----------------------------------------------------------------------------
  Random-effects Parameters  |   Estimate   Std. Err.    [95% Conf. Interval]
-----------------------------+-----------------------------------------------
region: Identity             |
                  var(_cons) |   1.07817   1.067804    .1547639    7.511127
-----------------------------+-----------------------------------------------
neighbourh~d: Unstructured   |
               var(activity) |   .0405534    .02266    .0135645    .1212417
                  var(_cons) |   137.5904  67.65923    52.48257    360.7125
          cov(activity,_cons)|  -2.360124   1.22754   -4.766057    .0458094
-----------------------------+-----------------------------------------------
                var(Residual)|   28.1099   1.629549    25.09081    31.49228
-----------------------------------------------------------------------------
LR test vs. linear model: chi2(4) = 54.69               Prob > chi2 = 0.0000
```

added to the model. As has been mentioned before, it is rather strange to assume that the random intercept and random slope on a particular level are independent.

To evaluate whether a random slope for activity on neighbourhood level must be added to the model, the likelihood ratio test can be performed. To do so, the -2 log likelihood of the model with two random intercepts has to be compared with the -2 log likelihood of the model shown in Output 2.9. The -2 log likelihood of the latter equals $-2 \times -2141.5435 = 4283.087$. The -2 log likelihood of the model with two random intercepts was 4293.7258. So, the difference between the two models equals 10.64. This difference follows a Chi-square distribution with two degrees of freedom – the variance of the slopes on neighbourhood level and the covariance between the random intercept and random slope on neighbourhood level – which is highly significant.

The last possibility for a random coefficient in the present model is allowing the regression coefficient for activity to differ between regions. When the analysis in which the intercepts as well as the slopes for activity were assumed to be random on both neighbourhood level and region level, an error message occurs. In this error message it is mentioned that there are problems with the Hessian matrix. In most situations, it is said that the 'Hessian matrix is not negative semidefinite.' Although this is a quite complicated mathematical issue, it basically means that no optimal solution for the likelihood function can be derived. There are several ways to deal with this problem. Most researchers will conclude that when there is no optimal solution it is better not to add the random slope for activity on region level to the model and report the results of the model with two random intercepts and a random slope for activity on neighbourhood level. Because activity is a continuous variable with values far above zero, another possibility is to use the centred variable for activity as the independent variable (see Section 2.5). Besides a better interpretation of the intercept and the random intercept variance, centring the independent variable also leads to less complicated estimates. When the same analysis is performed with the centred activity variable, there is no error message, but the iterations will never stop, also indicating that no optimal solution can be achieved. To stop the model endlessly iterating, a maximum number of iterations can be given. Output 2.10 shows the result of an analysis with a random intercept and random slope for activity (the centred variable) on both neighbourhood and region level and a maximum number of 50 iterations.

From Output 2.10 it can be seen that the estimation of the standard errors of the variances in the random part of the regression model lead to problems. It is therefore questionable whether the results of the analysis shown in Output 2.10 are valid. Another possibility to reach an optimal solution for the maximum-likelihood estimation is to increase the tolerance factor. When the log likelihood changes by a relative amount less than the tolerance factor, the optimal solution is derived. In some situations the optimal solution is not derived because the estimates jump between two possibilities for which the difference in log likelihood is slightly bigger than the tolerance factor. A slight increase in tolerance factor will sometimes lead to a proper solution. Output 2.11 shows the results of an analysis with a

Output 2.10 Result of a linear mixed model analysis of the relationship between physical activity and health, with a random intercept and random slope for activity (centred) on both neighbourhood and region level with a maximum number of 50 iterations

```
Mixed-effects ML regression                       Number of obs      =        684

-------------------------------------------------------------------------
                   |   No. of      Observations per Group
    Group Variable |   Groups   Minimum    Average   Maximum
-------------------+-----------------------------------------------------
            region |     12        22        57.0        84
      neighbourh~d |     48         4        14.3        49
-------------------------------------------------------------------------

                                                  Wald chi2(1)       =      69.80
Log likelihood = -2134.7689                       Prob > chi2        =     0.0000

-------------------------------------------------------------------------
       health |    Coef.    Std. Err.      z     P>|z|    [95% Conf. Interval]
--------------+----------------------------------------------------------
   activity_c~t |  .552686   .0661508     8.35   0.000    .4230327   .6823392
         _cons |  30.65911  .6135853    49.97   0.000    29.4565    31.86171
-------------------------------------------------------------------------


-------------------------------------------------------------------------
    Random-effects Parameters  |  Estimate  Std. Err.    [95% Conf. Interval]
-------------------------------+-----------------------------------------
region: Unstructured           |
             var(activi~t)     |  .0325799      .           .           .
             var(_cons)        |  3.547446      .           .           .
         cov(activi~t,_cons)   |  -.339964      .           .           .
-------------------------------+-----------------------------------------
neighbourh~d: Unstructured     |
             var(activi~t)     |  .0078474      .           .           .
             var(_cons)        |  1.221537      .           .           .
         cov(activi~t,_cons)   |  -.0952252     .           .           .
-------------------------------+-----------------------------------------
             var(Residual)     |  28.13156      .           .           .
-------------------------------------------------------------------------
LR test vs. linear model: chi2(6) = 68.24                Prob > chi2 = 0.0000
```

random intercept and random slope for activity (the centred variable) on both neighbourhood and region level with an increased tolerance factor.

When both alternative ways to obtain an optimal solution are compared to each other, it can be seen that the log likelihood values are exactly the same, that the regression coefficients in the fixed part of the regression model are exactly the same and that the estimates of the variance components are exactly the same. So, the results shown in Output 2.10 and Output 2.11 are probably valid. When the -2 log likelihood of het model with two random intercepts and two random slopes ($-2 \times -2134.7689 = 4269.5378$) is compared to the -2 log likelihood of the model with two random intercepts and only a random slope for activity on neighbourhood level

Output 2.11 Result of a linear mixed model analysis of the relationship between physical activity and health, with a random intercept and random slope for activity (centred) on both neighbourhood and region level with an increased tolerance factor

```
Mixed-effects ML regression                    Number of obs     =        684

                    |    No. of      Observations per Group
   Group Variable   |    Groups   Minimum    Average    Maximum
--------------------+------------------------------------------------
            region  |      12         22        57.0        84
       neighbourh~d |      48          4        14.3        49
--------------------------------------------------------------------

                                               Wald chi2(1)      =      69.85
Log likelihood = -2134.7689                    Prob > chi2       =     0.0000

--------------------------------------------------------------------------------
     health |     Coef.   Std. Err.      z     P>|z|    [95% Conf. Interval]
------------+-------------------------------------------------------------------
 activity_c~t |  .5526918   .0661286    8.36   0.000    .4230821    .6823015
       _cons |  30.65904   .6133467   49.99   0.000    29.4569    31.86117
--------------------------------------------------------------------------------


--------------------------------------------------------------------------------
  Random-effects Parameters   |   Estimate   Std. Err.    [95% Conf. Interval]
------------------------------+-------------------------------------------------
region: Unstructured          |
              var(activi~t)   |   .0325504   .0206541    .0093852    .1128929
              var(_cons)      |   3.543943   1.840462    1.280665    9.807037
         cov(activi~t,_cons)  |  -.3396419   .1795942   -.6916401    .0123563
------------------------------+-------------------------------------------------
neighbourh~d: Unstructured    |
              var(activi~t)   |    .00783    .0080374    .0010472    .0585467
              var(_cons)      |   1.22161    .8043092    .3361247    4.439811
         cov(activi~t,_cons)  |  -.0952675   .0818132   -.2556183    .0650834
------------------------------+-------------------------------------------------
              var(Residual)   |  28.13253   1.586327    25.18904    31.41999
--------------------------------------------------------------------------------
LR test vs. linear model: chi2(6) = 68.24              Prob > chi2 = 0.0000
```

(4283.087) it can be seen that this difference (evaluated on a Chi-square distribution with two degrees of freedom) is highly significant. Note that in this particular example the alternative ways to obtain an optimal solution only give a solution when the centred variable for activity is used. This is, however, no problem for the interpretation of the regression coefficient of interest, which is not influenced by centring a variable.

Thus, if it is believed that the alternative ways to obtain an optimal solution in this example are valid, the most appropriate estimate of the relationship between physical activity and health can be found in Output 2.10 and Output 2.11. The regression coefficient for activity is 0.55 and the corresponding 95% CI ranges from 0.42 to 0.68. The p-value of the relationship between physical activity and health is <0.001. It should, however, be realised that most researchers will report the results of the analysis with two random intercepts and a random slope for activity on neighbourhood level, the results shown in Output 2.9.

2.7 Assumptions in Mixed Model Analysis

Because linear mixed model analysis is an extension of standard linear regression analysis, all assumptions for standard linear regression analysis also hold for linear mixed model analysis. So, the continuous outcome variable should be normally distributed, i.e. the residuals should be normally distributed. As in standard linear regression analysis, this can be investigated by inspection of the distribution of the residuals. Moreover, the residuals should also be uncorrelated. In most mixed model studies this should not be a big problem, because the reason for performing a mixed model analysis in the first place is that there are correlated observations (i.e. correlated residuals) in the data to be analysed. Basically, by using mixed model analysis the problem of these correlated residuals is more or less solved. However, there are research situations in which the use of mixed model analysis only partly solves the problem of the correlated residuals. This is, for instance, sometimes the case in longitudinal studies (see Chapter 9).

An additional assumption that is typical for mixed model analysis was already mentioned in the earlier sections: the intercepts and slopes from which the variance is estimated must be more or less normally distributed. Whether or not this is a reasonable assumption can, for instance, be investigated by analysing the mean values of the outcome variable for the different groups (i.e. neighbourhoods). Figure 2.11 shows the distribution of the mean values of health for the 48 neighbourhoods in the present example.

From Figure 2.11 it can be seen that the distribution of the mean values of health for the different neighbourhoods is slightly skewed to the left. However, the skewness is not that strong, so it can be concluded that the assumption regarding the normal distribution of the intercepts holds.

In addition to checking the assumptions of the linear mixed model analysis, it can also be important to investigate whether the model coefficients are influenced by certain data-points or whether outliers are present

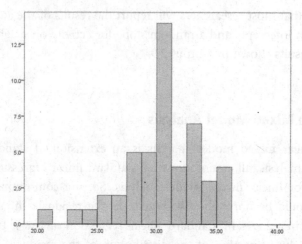

Figure 2.11 Distribution of the mean values of health of the different neighbourhoods in the example dataset.

in the analysed dataset. Because of the mixed model structure of the data, outliers (or influencing data points) can occur at different levels. Observations of subjects can influence the overall relationship that is analysed or can be outliers on subject level. On the other hand, a single observation can also be an outlier for the particular neighbourhood to whom that subjects belongs. In other words, the subject observation can be an outlier on neighbourhood level. For detailed information regarding outliers and influencing data-points in mixed model analysis, reference is made to Atkinson (1986), Barnett and Lewis (1994), Lawrence (1995) or Langford and Lewis (1998).

2.8 Comments

2.8.1 Which Regression Coefficients Can Be Assumed to Be Random?

In the present example, only one independent variable was included in the model (i.e. physical activity). Because physical activity was measured on subject level it was theoretically possible to add a random slope for activity on neighbourhood level and region level to the model. A general rule concerning random slopes is that they can only be considered to be random at a level above that on which they are measured. In the present example this means that because activity is measured on subject level, activity can only be

assumed to be random on the levels above subject level (i.e. on neighbourhood level and on region level). In line with this, if a variable was measured
on neighbourhood level, for instance the number of playing grounds in a
particular neighbourhood, the regression coefficient (i.e. slope) for that
particular variable can only be assumed to be random on region level.

2.8.2 Random Regression Coefficients versus Fixed Regression Coefficients

Within mixed model analysis the regression model is divided into a fixed
part and a random part. Therefore, a distinction can be made between fixed
and random coefficients. It should be realised that this distinction differs
from the distinction between random and fixed factors in the traditional
analysis of variance. In analysis of variance a random factor is defined as: 'a
categorical variable in which the groups are a random sample of all possible
groups about which conclusions are desired' (e.g. neighbourhood or
region). A fixed factor is defined as: 'a categorical variable about which
conclusions are desired for every group' (e.g. gender). In mixed model
analysis, however, a fixed regression coefficient is just the regression coefficient itself. In principle, all regression coefficients of a mixed model analysis
are fixed, because in general one is interested in the magnitude of the
regression coefficients. In addition to the fixed part of the regression
coefficient, each regression coefficient can also be considered to be random
(depending on the level on which the variable is measured [see Section
2.8.1]). This random part of the regression coefficient is the variation of the
regression coefficient between the groups considered (e.g. neighbourhoods,
regions, etc.). The term 'random' is probably not the most appropriate in
this respect, because the regression coefficients are not really random; they
are only assumed to be different for different groups.

2.8.3 Maximum Likelihood versus Restricted Maximum Likelihood

In all analyses performed so far in this chapter, the regression coefficients
and variances were estimated by maximum likelihood (ML). There is also
another procedure available that can be used to estimate the regression
coefficients and variances of a mixed model analysis, i.e. restricted maximum likelihood (REML). It should be noted that in most software packages the REML estimation procedure is the default (see also Chapter 13).

There is no real consensus concerning the best estimation procedure. It is often argued that REML is better for the estimation of random variances, while ML is better for the estimation of the (fixed) regression coefficients. In general, the (fixed) regression coefficients are of major interest; therefore, in the examples presented in this book, a ML estimation procedure is used. To illustrate the differences between the ML and the REML estimation procedure, the relationship between physical activity and health with both a random intercept and a random slope on neighbourhood level and a random intercept on region level was also estimated with REML. Output 2.12 shows the result of this analysis, while Table 2.2 summarises the results of both analyses.

From Table 2.2 it can be seen that the differences between the two estimation procedures are very small. Not surprisingly, the only differences

Output 2.12 Result of a linear mixed model analysis of the relationship between physical activity and health, with both a random intercept and a random slope for activity on neighbourhood level and with a random intercept on region level performed with restricted maximum likelihood

```
Mixed-effects REML regression                    Number of obs    =        684

----------------------------------------------------------------------
                   |  No. of       Observations per Group
 Group Variable    |  Groups    Minimum    Average    Maximum
-------------------+--------------------------------------------------
          region   |    12         22        57.0         84
    neighbourh~d   |    48          4        14.3         49
----------------------------------------------------------------------

                                            Wald chi2(1)     =      140.61
Log restricted-likelihood = -2143.5624      Prob > chi2      =      0.0000

----------------------------------------------------------------------
     health |    Coef.    Std. Err.      z     P>|z|    [95% Conf. Interval]
------------+---------------------------------------------------------
   activity |  .5817823   .0490628    11.86    0.000     .485621    .6779437
      _cons |  1.319233   2.653513     0.50    0.619    -3.881557   6.520024
----------------------------------------------------------------------


----------------------------------------------------------------------
  Random-effects Parameters   |   Estimate   Std. Err.    [95% Conf. Interval]
------------------------------+---------------------------------------
region: Identity              |
                 var(_cons)   |   1.353458   1.251563    .2209665    8.290167
------------------------------+---------------------------------------
neighbourh~d: Unstructured    |
              var(activity)   |   .0429372   .0235545    .0146515    .1258303
                 var(_cons)   |   142.0153   69.54347    54.38889    370.8173
        cov(activity,_cons)   |  -2.465611   1.268865   -4.95254     .0213183
------------------------------+---------------------------------------
              var(Residual)   |   28.11291   1.630417    25.09228    31.49717
----------------------------------------------------------------------
LR test vs. linear model: chi2(4) = 56.53            Prob > chi2 = 0.0000
```

Table 2.2 Relationship between activity and health, estimated with a maximum-likelihood (ML) estimation procedure and with a restricted maximum-likelihood (REML) procedure

	ML estimate	REML estimate
Intercept	30.49 (0.45)	30.50 (0.47)
Activity random intercept	0.58 (0.05)	0.58 (0.05)
On neighbourhood level random slope for activity	2.85 (1.74)	2.69 (1.70)
On neighbourhood level random intercept	0.04 (0.02)	0.04 (0.02)
On region level	1.08 (1.07)	1.35 (1.25)
Log likelihood	−2141.5	−2143.6

were observed for the variance of the random intercepts and the $-2\log$ likelihood. So, the discussion about whether maximum likelihood or restricted maximum likelihood should be used for mixed model analyses is basically irrelevant. It should furthermore be noted that for restricted maximum-likelihood estimation the likelihood is totally based on the estimation of the variances in the random part of the model. Thus, when the likelihood ratio test is used for evaluating whether a particular variable should be added to the fixed part of the model, the likelihood estimated with restricted maximum likelihood is not valid and can therefore not be used (Morrell, 1998; Oehlert, 2012).

3

What Is Gained by Using Mixed Model Analysis?

3.1 Introduction

Before mixed model analysis was developed, the problem of correlated observations within neighbourhoods, medical doctors, schools, etc. was tackled in two ways: either ignoring the fact that the observations are correlated or combining the correlated observations into one value. In fact, both methods are still frequently used. Ignoring the fact that the observations are correlated indicates that all observations are analysed as independent. In Chapter 2, this method was called naive analysis, but it is also referred to as disaggregation analysis. The other possibility is not to ignore the dependency of the observations, but to analyse the group observations instead of the individual observations. In order to do this some sort of average value of the observations for each group must first be calculated, and then these averages can be used as outcome in a standard regression analysis. This method is referred to as aggregation analysis. To answer the question of what is gained by using mixed model analysis, it is interesting to compare the results obtained from these three types of analyses: the naive/disaggregation analysis, the aggregation analysis and the (more sophisticated) mixed model analysis.

3.2 Example with a Balanced Dataset

In the first example, a dataset from a randomised controlled trial (RCT) is used, and the outcome variable in this RCT is a continuous health outcome. The total study population consists of 200 patients, randomly divided into an intervention group and a control group. The intervention was performed by 20 general practitioners (GPs), and in this balanced dataset each GP had 10 patients. The randomisation was performed on patient level, which means that for each GP half of the patients were allocated to the intervention group and the other half to the control group. Table 3.1 shows descriptive information regarding the dataset that is used in this example.

The first analysis that was performed was a naive/disaggregation analysis or, in other words, all patients are considered to be independent. Output 3.1 shows the result of this analysis. The regression coefficient is exactly the same as the regression coefficient obtained from a standard linear regression analysis. To illustrate this, Output 3.2 shows the output of a standard linear regression analysis. The only difference is that in standard linear regression analysis the regression coefficients are estimated with ordinary least squares (OLS), while with mixed model analysis the regression coefficients are estimated with maximum likelihood. As a consequence of this difference, in standard linear regression analysis a t-statistic and a t-distribution are used to evaluate whether or not the effect of the

Table 3.1 Descriptive information regarding the example dataset

	Mean	Standard deviation
Health	6.65	0.87
	Percentage	
Intervention (no/yes)	50%/50%	

Output 3.1 Result of a naive linear mixed analysis performed on a balanced dataset to determine the effect of the intervention on a certain health outcome without adjusting for GP

```
Mixed-effects ML regression                    Number of obs      =         200
                                               Wald chi2(1)       =        5.76
Log likelihood = -251.84924                    Prob > chi2        =      0.0164

------------------------------------------------------------------------------
    health |      Coef.   Std. Err.      z    P>|z|     [95% Conf. Interval]
-----------+------------------------------------------------------------------
intervention |    .2892   .1205484     2.40   0.016     .0529294    .5254705
      _cons |    6.5013   .0852406    76.27   0.000     6.334231    6.668369
------------------------------------------------------------------------------

------------------------------------------------------------------------------
  Random-effects Parameters |   Estimate   Std. Err.     [95% Conf. Interval]
----------------------------+-------------------------------------------------
              var(Residual) |   .726596    .0726596       .597273    .8839204
------------------------------------------------------------------------------
```

Output 3.2 Result of an OLS linear regression analysis performed on a balanced dataset to determine the effect of the intervention on a certain health outcome

```
      Source |       SS           df       MS           Number of obs   =       200
-------------+----------------------------------        F(1, 198)       =      5.70
       Model |  4.18183188          1   4.18183188       Prob > F        =    0.0179
    Residual |  145.319205        198    .73393538       R-squared       =    0.0280
-------------+----------------------------------        Adj R-squared   =    0.0231
       Total |  149.501037        199   .751261493       Root MSE        =    .8567


--------------------------------------------------------------------------------
      health |      Coef.   Std. Err.      t    P>|t|     [95% Conf. Interval]
-------------+------------------------------------------------------------------
intervention |      .2892   .1211557     2.39   0.018     .0502788     .5281212
       _cons |     6.5013    .08567     75.89   0.000     6.332357     6.670243
--------------------------------------------------------------------------------
```

intervention is significant and to estimate the 95% confidence interval (CI). With mixed model analysis, on the other hand, this is done with the z-test and the standard normal distribution. Besides that, it can be seen that the magnitude of the standard error is slightly bigger when obtained from an OLS regression.

From Output 3.1 and Output 3.2 it can be seen that the intervention effect is 0.289, with a standard error of 0.121. Based on the mixed model analysis, the 95% CI of this intervention effect ranges from 0.053 to 0.525. Output 3.3 shows the results of the mixed model analysis, not ignoring the dependency of the observations. In the mixed model analysis, both a random intercept and a random slope for the intervention variable were modelled.

When a mixed model analysis is performed with both a random intercept and a random slope for the intervention variable, the intervention effect remains exactly the same (i.e. 0.289), but the standard error increases from 0.121 to 0.175 (see Output 3.1 and Output 3.3). The 95% CI around the intervention effect estimated with a mixed model analysis is therefore wider and ranges from −0.054 to 0.633, which is no longer significant. The fact that the standard error obtained from the mixed model analysis is higher than the standard error obtained from the naive/disaggregated analysis is not surprising. In the analysis that ignores the dependency of the observations, each observation is considered to provide 100% new information. In a mixed model analysis, an adjustment is made for GP, which means that the information provided by a patient belonging to the same GP does not give 100% new information but less. So, because the total amount of information used in a mixed model analysis is less than in a naive/disaggregated analysis

Output 3.3 Result of a linear mixed model analysis performed on a balanced dataset to determine the effect of the intervention on a certain health outcome with both a random intercept and a random slope for the intervention on GP level

```
Mixed-effects ML regression                      Number of obs     =        200
Group variable: gp                               Number of groups  =         20

                                                 Obs per group:
                                                              min =         10
                                                              avg =       10.0
                                                              max =         10

                                                 Wald chi2(1)      =       2.72
Log likelihood = -224.28932                      Prob > chi2       =     0.0989

------------------------------------------------------------------------------
      health |     Coef.   Std. Err.      z    P>|z|     [95% Conf. Interval]
-------------+----------------------------------------------------------------
intervention |    .2892    .1752275     1.65   0.099    -.0542396    .6326396
       _cons |   6.5013    .1104318    58.87   0.000     6.284858    6.717742
------------------------------------------------------------------------------

------------------------------------------------------------------------------
  Random-effects Parameters  |   Estimate   Std. Err.     [95% Conf. Interval]
-----------------------------+------------------------------------------------
gp: Unstructured             |
           var(interv~n)     |   .4493851   .1950646      .1919276    1.052204
             var(_cons)      |   .1615493   .0776767      .0629546    .4145555
       cov(interv~n,_cons)   |  -.0714165   .0935736     -.2548174    .1119844
-----------------------------+------------------------------------------------
             var(Residual)   |   .4117709   .0460374      .3307413    .5126523
------------------------------------------------------------------------------
LR test vs. linear model: chi2(3) = 55.12              Prob > chi2 = 0.0000
```

the standard error of the estimate will be higher. The magnitude of the new information provided by each individual patient depends on the magnitude of the intraclass correlation coefficient (ICC; see Section 2.3). The higher the ICC, the less new information is provided by a patient belonging to the same GP, and the higher the standard error estimated with mixed model analysis will be compared to the standard error estimated with a naive/ disaggregation analysis.

When the analysis is performed on the average health outcomes of the patients of the 20 medical doctors (see Output 3.4a and Output 3.4b), it can be seen that the regression coefficient of this aggregation analysis is exactly the same as for the other two analyses. However, because only 40 observations are analysed (i.e. the average values of the intervention patients and the average value of the control patients of the 20 GPs), the standard error of the regression coefficient is higher than in the other 2 analyses. From Output 3.4a and Output 3.4b it can also be seen that, again, the standard error obtained from an OLS regression analysis is higher than the standard

Output 3.4a Result of an aggregated (on GP level) mixed model analysis performed on a balanced dataset to determine the effect of the intervention on a certain health outcome

```
Mixed-effects ML regression                    Number of obs    =        40
                                               Wald chi2(1)     =      2.11
Log likelihood = -38.290189                    Prob > chi2      =    0.1467
------------------------------------------------------------------------------
    health1 |   Coef.    Std. Err.     z    P>|z|    [95% Conf. Interval]
------------+-----------------------------------------------------------------
intervention |   .2892   .1992936    1.45   0.147   -.1014082    .6798082
       _cons |  6.5013   .1409218   46.13   0.000    6.225098    6.777502
------------------------------------------------------------------------------

------------------------------------------------------------------------------
Random-effects Parameters  |  Estimate   Std. Err.   [95% Conf. Interval]
---------------------------+--------------------------------------------------
             var(Residual) |  .3971792    .088812     .256243     .6156317
------------------------------------------------------------------------------
```

Output 3.4b Result of an aggregated (on GP level) OLS linear regression analysis performed on a balanced dataset to determine the effect of the intervention on a certain health outcome

```
    Source |       SS          df       MS        Number of obs   =       40
-----------+--------------------------------       F(1, 38)        =     2.00
     Model |  .8363664          1    .8363664      Prob > F        =   0.1654
  Residual | 15.8871692         38   .4180834      R-squared       =   0.0500
-----------+--------------------------------       Adj R-squared   =   0.0250
     Total | 16.7235356         39   .428808605    Root MSE        =   .64659

------------------------------------------------------------------------------
    health1 |   Coef.    Std. Err.     t    P>|t|    [95% Conf. Interval]
------------+-----------------------------------------------------------------
intervention |   .2892   .2044709    1.41   0.165   -.1247297    .7031297
       _cons |  6.5013   .1445827   44.97   0.000    6.208608    6.793992
------------------------------------------------------------------------------
```

error obtained from a maximum likelihood estimation procedure and that the differences between the two methods is bigger than the differences observed in the naive/disaggregated analyses. The reason for this is the smaller sample size in the aggregated analyses. For relatively big sample sizes the standard errors obtained from both methods will be more or less the same.

When the regression coefficients and standard errors were estimated with restricted maximum likelihood (REML) instead of maximum likelihood, the standard error will be exactly the same as the standard error obtained from an OLS regression analysis (see Output 3.4c). For the discussion around maximum likelihood estimations and restricted maximum likelihood estimations see Section 2.8.3.

Output 3.4c Result of an aggregated (on GP level) mixed model analysis performed on a balanced dataset to determine the effect of the intervention on a certain health outcome performed with REML

```
Mixed-effects REML regression              Number of obs    =        40

                                           Wald chi2(1)     =      2.00
Log restricted-likelihood = -40.345984     Prob > chi2      =    0.1572

-----------------------------------------------------------------------
   health1 |    Coef.   Std. Err.      z    P>|z|    [95% Conf. Interval]
-----------+-----------------------------------------------------------
intervention |    .2892   .2044709    1.41   0.157   -.1115556    .6899556
      _cons |   6.5013   .1445827   44.97   0.000    6.217923    6.784677
-----------------------------------------------------------------------


-----------------------------------------------------------------------
 Random-effects Parameters  |  Estimate   Std. Err.    [95% Conf. Interval]
----------------------------+------------------------------------------
               var(Residual) |  .4180834   .0934863     .2697295    .6480334
-----------------------------------------------------------------------
```

3.3 Example with an Unbalanced Dataset

The differences between a naive/disaggregation analysis, a mixed model analysis, and an aggregation analysis are different when the dataset is unbalanced. In the following example the dataset used in the example in Section 3.2 is changed in such a way that for half of the GPs, only eight patients are included in the study. For five GPs, three patients are allocated to the intervention group and five patients to the control group, while for the other five GPs, three patients were allocated to the control group and five patients to the intervention group. So, instead of 200 patients in the earlier example, this dataset includes 180 patients. Output 3.5 shows the results of the analysis ignoring the dependency of the observations within the GPs (i.e. the results of the naive/disaggregation analysis).

From Output 3.5 it can be seen that the intervention effect is 0.351, with a standard error of 0.127. This results in a 95% CI, ranging from 0.101 to 0.601; the corresponding p-value is 0.006. When a mixed model analysis is performed (again with both a random intercept and a random slope for the intervention variable), not only is the standard error of the intervention effect different, but the intervention effect itself is as well (see Output 3.6). The intervention effect is now 0.358, with a 95% CI ranging from -0.010 to 0.727, and the p-value for this intervention effect, is 0.056.

When an aggregation analysis is applied to this unbalanced dataset, both the intervention effect and the corresponding standard error are different from the results of the previous analyses (see Output 3.7).

Output 3.5 Result of a naive linear mixed model analysis performed on an unbalanced dataset to determine the effect of the intervention on a certain health outcome without adjusting for GP

```
Mixed-effects ML regression                          Number of obs     =        180

                                                     Wald chi2(1)      =       7.59
Log likelihood =  -227.1465                          Prob > chi2       =     0.0059

-------------------------------------------------------------------------------------
      health |      Coef.   Std. Err.      z    P>|z|     [95% Conf. Interval]
-------------+-----------------------------------------------------------------------
intervention |    .3511111     .12741    2.76   0.006     .101392     .6008302
       _cons |    6.445444   .0900925   71.54   0.000    6.268866    6.622022
-------------------------------------------------------------------------------------


-------------------------------------------------------------------------------------
Random-effects Parameters   |   Estimate   Std. Err.     [95% Conf. Interval]
----------------------------+--------------------------------------------------------
               var(Residual) |   .7304992   .0770014     .5941488     .8981405
-------------------------------------------------------------------------------------
```

Output 3.6 Result of a linear mixed model analysis performed on a unbalanced dataset to determine the effect of the intervention on a certain health outcome with both a random intercept and a random slope for the intervention on GP level

```
Mixed-effects ML regression                          Number of obs     =        180
Group variable: gp                                   Number of groups  =         20

                                                     Obs per group:
                                                                  min =          8
                                                                  avg =        9.0
                                                                  max =         10

                                                     Wald chi2(1)      =       3.64
Log likelihood = -202.24904                          Prob > chi2       =     0.0564

-------------------------------------------------------------------------------------
      health |      Coef.   Std. Err.      z    P>|z|     [95% Conf. Interval]
-------------+-----------------------------------------------------------------------
intervention |    .3584268    .187884    1.91   0.056    -.0098191     .7266726
       _cons |    6.469326   .1075293   60.16   0.000    6.258572    6.680079
-------------------------------------------------------------------------------------


-------------------------------------------------------------------------------------
Random-effects Parameters   |   Estimate   Std. Err.     [95% Conf. Interval]
----------------------------+--------------------------------------------------------
gp: Unstructured             |
           var(interv~n)     |   .5179796   .2194353     .2257939    1.188265
             var(_cons)      |   .1379199    .07271      .0490774    .3875895
        cov(interv~n,_cons)  |  -.0861715   .0962636    -.2748448    .1025017
----------------------------+--------------------------------------------------------
               var(Residual) |   .4093401   .0486792     .3242338    .5167854
-------------------------------------------------------------------------------------
LR test vs. linear model: chi2(3) = 49.79                   Prob > chi2 = 0.0000
```

Output 3.7 Result of an aggregation (at GP level) mixed model analysis performed on an unbalanced dataset to determine the effect of the intervention on a certain health outcome

```
Mixed-effects ML regression                    Number of obs    =         40

                                               Wald chi2(1)     =       3.12
Log likelihood = -38.130086                    Prob > chi2      =     0.0775

--------------------------------------------------------------------------------
average_hea~h |     Coef.   Std. Err.      z    P>|z|     [95% Conf. Interval]
--------------+-----------------------------------------------------------------
 intervention |    .35042   .1984975     1.77   0.078    -.0386279    .7394679
        _cons |   6.48548   .1403589    46.21   0.000     6.210382    6.760578
--------------------------------------------------------------------------------


--------------------------------------------------------------------------------
Random-effects Parameters  |   Estimate   Std. Err.     [95% Conf. Interval]
---------------------------+----------------------------------------------------
          var(Residual)  |   .3940124   .0881039         .2542     .6107232
--------------------------------------------------------------------------------
```

3.4 Cluster Randomisation

The examples described in Sections 3.2 and 3.3 are related to a randomisation at patient level. This means that in the mixed model analysis the intervention effect can also be considered random among GPs, meaning it was possible to assume a random slope for the intervention variable. When a cluster randomisation design is used, so when the randomisation is not carried out on patient level, but on GP level, the intervention effect cannot be considered to be random among the GPs. This is based on the rule that random slopes can only be considered on a level above the level on which the specific variable is measured. However, the differences and equalities between a naive/disaggregation analysis, a mixed model analysis and an aggregation analysis are comparable to the differences described for a dataset in which the randomisation is carried out on patient level. Table 3.2 summarises the results of the three different types of analyses on the dataset with cluster randomisation.

3.5 Comments

Irrespective of the way in which randomisation is performed (either on patient level or on GP level), the differences between a naive/disaggregation analysis, a mixed model analysis and an aggregation analysis depend on

Table 3.2 Results of a naive/disaggregation analysis, a mixed model analysis and an aggregation analysis on a dataset in which a cluster randomisation is performed, i.e. the randomisation is carried out on GP level

	Intervention effect	Standard error	p-value
Balanced dataset[1]			
naive/disaggregation	0.259	0.121	0.032
mixed model analysis	0.259	0.213	0.224
aggregation	0.259	0.225	0.265
Unbalanced dataset[2]			
naive/disaggregation	0.242	0.129	0.061
mixed model analysis	0.257	0.215	0.231
aggregation	0.269	0.216	0.213

[1] In the balanced dataset 200 patients were included, equally divided among the 20 GPs.
[2] In the unbalanced dataset, for half of the GPs only eight patients were included, resulting in a total of 180 patients.

whether or not the dataset is balanced. If the dataset is balanced, the only difference between the methods is observed in the standard error of the intervention effect. However, when the dataset is unbalanced, there is not only a difference in the standard errors but there is also a difference in the estimated intervention effect between the three methods. The reason why the intervention effect is only different for an unbalanced dataset has to do with the possible confounding influence of the group variable on the intervention effect. A confounder has to be related to both the outcome variable and the independent variable, which is not the case in a balanced dataset. Because in a balanced dataset the intervention variable is not related to the group variable, the group variable cannot influence the magnitude of the intervention effect. When the dataset is unbalanced, however, the intervention variable is related to the group variable and, therefore, the group variable can be a confounder in the estimation of the intervention effect. Because of that, the intervention effect is different between the three methods when obtained on a unbalanced dataset.

4

Logistic Mixed Model Analysis

4.1 Introduction

In the foregoing chapters, mixed model analysis was explained with examples from studies with continuous outcome variables (i.e. linear mixed model analysis). One of the biggest advantages of mixed model analysis is that it can be used for the analysis of dichotomous outcome variables as well (i.e. logistic mixed model analysis). The general principles behind a logistic mixed model analysis are the same as those described in Chapter 2 for a linear mixed model analysis. So, in general, mixed model analysis with a dichotomous outcome variable is a logistic regression analysis in which an additional, very efficient, adjustment can be made for categorical variables with many groups, such as neighbourhood, general practitioner or school. It should be realised that within a logistic mixed model analysis the estimation of the random variances, in particular, is mathematically quite difficult and that different software packages use different estimation procedures. Unfortunately, these different procedures often lead to different results. See Section 4.4 for further information about the use of different estimation procedures and Chapter 13 for a comparison between software packages.

4.2 Example

The use of a logistic mixed model analysis can best be illustrated by analysing an example dataset. The dataset is the same as was used in the example with continuous outcome variables; the only difference is that now a dichotomous health indicator is used as outcome dividing the subjects into relatively bad health and relatively good health. Again the relationship

Table 4.1 Descriptive information regarding the example dataset

	Mean	Standard deviation
Physical activity	50.2	5.8
	Percentage	
Health (bad/good)	46.1%/53.9%	

Output 4.1 Result of a naive logistic mixed model analysis of the relationship between physical activity and the dichotomous health indicator without an adjustment for neighbourhood

```
Logistic regression                            Number of obs    =         684

                                               Wald chi2(1)     =       88.56
Log likelihood = -417.26989                    Prob > chi2      =      0.0000
-------------------------------------------------------------------------------
health_dich |     Coef.   Std. Err.      z    P>|z|     [95% Conf. Interval]
------------+------------------------------------------------------------------
   activity |   .1550478   .0164762    9.41   0.000      .122755    .1873405
      _cons |  -7.605014   .8287765   -9.18   0.000    -9.229386   -5.980641
-------------------------------------------------------------------------------
```

between physical activity and health is analysed. Table 4.1 shows descriptive information regarding the dataset used in the example.

As can be seen from Table 4.1, almost half of the subjects were classified with either bad or good health. Because the same dataset is used as in Chapter 2, the subjects are living in 48 different neighbourhoods.

Output 4.1 shows the results of a naive logistic regression analysis of the relationship between physical activity and the dichotomous health indicator. In this first analysis all observations are assumed to be independent, i.e. no adjustment is made for neighbourhood.

Comparable to the output of a naive linear mixed model analysis, the first part of Output 4.1 shows some general information of the data (684 observations), the log likelihood of the model and the Chi-square test for all the variables in the model, which, again, is only the variable activity. The next part of the output contains the fixed part of the regression model with the regression coefficients, corresponding standard errors, z-values, p-values and the 95% confidence intervals (CI).

From Output 4.1 it can be seen that the regression coefficient for physical activity equals 0.1550478. The coefficient indicates the difference in the outcome of the logistic regression analysis (the natural log of the odds of being healthy) for a one unit difference in activity. In general this regression coefficient is transformed into an odds ratio by taking the e-power of the coefficient. In the example the odds ratio for physical activity is therefore EXP[0.155] = 1.168. This means that a difference of one unit in physical activity is associated with a 1.168 times higher odds to have good health. In the same way the 95% CI around the odds ratio can be calculated: EXP[regression coefficient $\pm$ 1.96 times the standard error]. In the present example the 95% CI around the odds ratio of 1.168 ranges between 1.131 and 1.206. This is a relatively small odds ratio with a narrow interval, which is due to the fact that it reflects the odds ratio related to only one unit difference in physical activity. The corresponding p-value can be found directly in the output and is <0.001. It is also possible to get the odds ratio and the corresponding 95% CI directly in the output (see Output 4.2).

Different from the results of the naive linear mixed model analysis, in the naive logistic mixed model analysis there is no random part of the regression model containing the residual variance. This has to do with the fact that a logistic regression analysis does not have a residual variance. Basically, in a logistic model the probability of having the outcome is modelled and this probability is modelled without error. The error in the estimation is outside the model in the comparison between the probability and the observed outcome which is either 0 or 1.

Output 4.3 shows the result of a logistic mixed model analysis in which an adjustment is made for the neighbourhood, or, in other words, a logistic mixed model with a random intercept on neighbourhood level.

The output of a logistic mixed model analysis is comparable to the output of a linear mixed model analysis. First some general information is

Output 4.2 Result of a naive logistic mixed model analysis of the relationship between physical activity and the dichotomous health indicator without an adjustment for neighbourhood with the effect estimate expressed as an odds ratio

```
Logistic regression                         Number of obs    =        684

                                            Wald chi2(1)     =      88.56
Log likelihood = -417.26989                 Prob > chi2      =     0.0000
-----------------------------------------------------------------------------
health_dich | Odds Ratio   Std. Err.      z    P>|z|     [95% Conf. Interval]
------------+----------------------------------------------------------------
   activity |   1.167714   .0192395     9.41   0.000      1.130607    1.206038
      _cons |   .0004979   .0004127    -9.18   0.000      .0000981    .0025272
-----------------------------------------------------------------------------
```

Output 4.3 Result of a logistic mixed model analysis of the relationship between physical activity and the dichotomous health indicator with a random intercept on neighbourhood level

```
Mixed-effects logistic regression          Number of obs    =        684
Group variable:     neighbourhood          Number of groups =         48

                                           Obs per group:
                                                        min =          4
                                                        avg =       14.3
                                                        max =         49

Integration method: mvaghermite             Integration pts. =         7

                                           Wald chi2(1)     =      83.43
Log likelihood = -408.96783                Prob > chi2      =     0.0000
-------------------------------------------------------------------------------
  health_dich |     Coef.   Std. Err.      z    P>|z|    [95% Conf. Interval]
--------------+----------------------------------------------------------------
     activity |  .1685528   .0184534     9.13   0.000    .1323849    .2047207
        _cons | -8.243316   .9319357    -8.85   0.000   -10.06988   -6.416756
--------------+----------------------------------------------------------------
neighbourhood |
    var(_cons)|  .4866812   .2171715                     .2029613    1.167013
-------------------------------------------------------------------------------
LR test vs. logistic model: chibar2(01) = 16.60        Prob >= chibar2 = 0.0000
```

provided. It can be seen that a mixed-effects logistic regression is performed and that the group variable is the neighbourhood. Furthermore, Output 4.3 shows that there are 684 observations and that there are 48 neighbourhoods. The number of subjects within a neighbourhood varies between 4 and 49. The output also shows the log likelihood and the integration method (*mvaghermite*). The latter stands for mean-variance adaptive Gauss–Hermite quadrature. It is a complicated method to calculate the log likelihood. See, for instance, Liu and Pierce (1994), Lesaffre and Spiessens (2001), Rabe-Hesketh et al. (2002), Skrondal and Rabe-Hesketh (2004) or Rabe-Hesketh et al. (2005) for mathematical details about this method.

The second part of Output 4.3 contains the (fixed) regression coefficient which is 0.1685528 for activity. As has been mentioned before, the coefficient indicates the difference in the natural log of the odds of being healthy for a one unit difference in activity. In general this regression coefficient is transformed into an odds ratio by taking the e-power of the coefficient. In this case the odds ratio for a one unit difference in activity to be healthy is 1.18. Also, for logistic mixed model analysis it is possible to get the odds ratio directly in the output. Output 4.4 shows the result of the logistic mixed model analysis with a random intercept on neighbourhood level, reporting odds ratios.

Output 4.4 Result of a logistic mixed model analysis of the relationship between physical activity and the dichotomous health indicator with a random intercept on neighbourhood level with the effect estimate expressed as an odds ratio

```
Mixed-effects logistic regression              Number of obs    =        684
Group variable:    neighbourhood               Number of groups =         48

                                               Obs per group:
                                                            min =          4
                                                            avg =       14.3
                                                            max =         49

Integration method: mvaghermite                Integration pts. =          7

                                               Wald chi2(1)     =      83.43
Log likelihood = -408.96783                    Prob > chi2      =     0.0000
-------------------------------------------------------------------------------
health_dich | Odds Ratio   Std. Err.      z    P>|z|     [95% Conf. Interval]
------------+------------------------------------------------------------------
   activity |  1.183591    .0218412     9.13   0.000     1.141548    1.227182
      _cons |  .000263     .0002451    -8.85   0.000     .0000423    .0016339
------------+------------------------------------------------------------------
neighbourh~d |
   var(_cons)|  .4866812    .2171715                     .2029613    1.167013
-------------------------------------------------------------------------------
LR test vs. logistic model: chibar2(01) = 16.60    Prob >= chibar2 = 0.0000
```

From Output 4.4 it can be seen that the odds ratio for physical activity is 1.18 and that the 95% CI ranges from 1.14 to 1.23; the corresponding p-value is <0.001.

The last part of Output 4.4 shows the random part of the regression model. It can be seen that the random intercept variance is equal to 0.4866812. As has been mentioned before, the logistic model does not have a residual variance.

To evaluate the necessity of adding a random intercept to the model, the likelihood ratio test can be applied. To do so, the $-2\log$ likelihood of the model without the random intercept (the naive logistic regression model) has to be compared with the $-2\log$ likelihood of the model with a random intercept. The $-2\log$ likelihood of the model without a random intercept (see Output 4.2) is $-2 \times -417.26989 = 834.54$, while the $-2\log$ likelihood of the model with a random intercept is $-2 \times -408.96783 = 817.94$. The difference between the two (16.6) follows a Chi-square distribution with one degree of freedom and is therefore highly significant. In other words, it is necessary to add a random intercept on neighbourhood level to the model.

The comparison of the $-2\log$ likelihood of the model with a random intercept and the naive logistic regression analysis can also be seen in the last line of the output, which gives the result of the likelihood ratio test to compare the two models with each other. The last line of the output shows the difference in $-2\log$ likelihood between the two models (16.6) and the corresponding p-value.

Looking at the magnitude of the relationship between physical activity and the dichotomous health indicator, it can be seen that both the regression coefficient and the standard error have increased compared to the results of a naive logistic regression analysis which were reported in Output 4.1. It was already mentioned in Chapter 3 that the increase in standard error when an adjustment is made for neighbourhood has to do with the fact that a subject living in the same neighbourhood does not provide 100% new information. Because in the naive analysis it is assumed that the observations of each subject are independent, all observations provide 100% new information. The difference between the regression coefficients has to do with actual confounding by neighbourhood (see Chapter 3). The next step in the modelling is to evaluate whether or not it is necessary to allow the relationship between physical activity and health to be different for the neighbourhoods. Or in other words, whether or not it is necessary to add a random slope for physical activity to the model. When the analysis is performed in the regular way, the model unfortunately does not converge. This was already seen in an earlier analysis (see Section 2.6). One possibility to deal with this problem is to use the centred value of physical activity instead of the original variable. Output 4.5 shows the result of the logistic mixed model analysis in which, in addition to a random intercept, a random slope for activity is considered and in which the centred value of activity is used as independent variable.

Based on Output 4.5, a likelihood ratio test can be performed to evaluate whether a random slope for activity on a neighbourhood level is necessary. The $-2\log$ likelihood of the model with both a random intercept and a random slope (and the covariance between the random intercept and random slope) is $-2 \times -408.45993 = 816.92$. The difference with the $-2\log$ likelihood of the model with only a random intercept is $817.94 - 816.92 = 1.02$, which follows a Chi-square distribution with two degrees of freedom and is therefore not statistically significant. In other words, a random slope for physical activity on neighbourhood level is not necessary, and the final logistic mixed model is a model with only a random intercept.

Output 4.5 Result of a logistic mixed model analysis of the relationship between physical activity (centred) and the dichotomous health indicator with a random intercept and random slope for activity on neighbourhood level

```
Mixed-effects logistic regression           Number of obs      =        684
Group variable:    neighbourhood            Number of groups   =         48

                                            Obs per group:
                                                         min =          4
                                                         avg =       14.3
                                                         max =         49

Integration method: mvaghermite             Integration pts.   =          7

                                            Wald chi2(1)       =      68.57
Log likelihood = -408.45993                 Prob > chi2        =     0.0000
------------------------------------------------------------------------------
 health_dich |     Coef.   Std. Err.      z    P>|z|    [95% Conf. Interval]
-------------+----------------------------------------------------------------
  activity_c~t |   .171361   .0206947    8.28   0.000    .1308002    .2119218
        _cons |  .1893429   .1437217    1.32   0.188   -.0923465    .4710323
-------------+----------------------------------------------------------------
neighbourh~d |
var(activi~t)|  .0010688   .0035978                    1.46e-06    .7837082
   var(_cons)|  .5191823   .2332014                    .2152709    1.252145
-------------+----------------------------------------------------------------
neighbourh~d |
   cov(_cons,|
  activity_c~t)|  -.0176314   .0197326   -0.89   0.372   -.0563066    .0210438
------------------------------------------------------------------------------
LR test vs. logistic model: chi2(3) = 17.62            Prob > chi2 = 0.0005
```

4.3 Intraclass Correlation Coefficient in Logistic Mixed Model Analysis

For continuous outcome variables it was mentioned that the dependency of the observations on a certain level could be estimated by the intraclass correlation coefficient (ICC) (see Section 2.3). The ICC was estimated as the ratio of the between-group variance and the total variance. Because the total variance is not directly available in a logistic model, an alternative way of estimating the ICC is provided by Eq. 4.1.

$$ICC = \frac{\sigma^2_{between}}{\sigma^2_{between} + \pi^2/3}$$

(4.1)

where $\sigma^2_{between}$ = between-group variance and $\pi = 3.14$.

The between-group variance provided in Output 4.3 can be used to estimate the ICC in the present example.

$$ICC = \frac{0.49}{0.49 + (3.14)^2/3} = 0.13$$

Although it is possible to estimate the ICC in a logistic mixed model analysis, it is questionable whether this should be done, mainly because a correlation coefficient for a dichotomous variable is very difficult to interpret. It is, therefore, also suggested that a so-called median odds ratio can be used as an alternative to the ICC for logistic mixed models (Larsen et al., 2000). The theory behind the median odds ratio sounds reasonable, but in practice it is not widely used.

For a more detailed mathematical explanation of logistic mixed model analysis, reference is made to Goldstein (2003).

4.4 Different Estimation Procedures

It was already mentioned that it is rather difficult to estimate the random variances in a logistic mixed model analysis, in particular. Therefore, many different estimation procedures are available. It should be realised that different software programs use different estimation procedures and that, even within software programs, different estimation procedures are available. It should furthermore be noted that the different estimation procedures can lead to markedly different results. The situation is even more complex, because it is not really clear which of the estimation procedures provides the most valid results. The results of a logistic mixed model analysis should, therefore, be interpreted with caution. A comparison between different software packages is provided in Chapter 13 (Section 13.4.3), and for detailed (mostly mathematical) discussion about the different estimation procedures for logistic mixed model analysis reference is made to Nelder and Lee (1992), Rodriguez and Goldman (1995, 1997, 2001), Goldstein and Rasbash (1996), Neuhaus and Lesparance (1996), Engel (1998), Moerbeek et al. (2001, 2003a) and Rabe-Hesketh et al. (2005).

4.5 Other Ways to Adjust for the Correlated Observations

Besides mixed model analysis, there are other methods available that can be used to take into account correlated observations or, in other words, that can adjust for a categorical variable with many groups in a very efficient way. One method which is often used in medical and epidemiological studies is generalised estimating equations (GEE). The difference between mixed model analysis and GEE analysis is the way in which the adjustment (for the categorical variable with many groups) is performed. It was already mentioned that within mixed model analysis the adjustment is performed by estimating the variance between the groups. Within GEE analysis this adjustment is performed by modelling the correlation within the groups. Without going into much detail, within GEE analysis a specific correlation structure has to be defined before analysis. Several options are available regarding the correlation structure. By far the most used correlation structure is the exchangeable structure, in which one average correlation over the groups is used to adjust for the dependency of the observations within the groups. We have already seen in Section 2.3, where the ICC was calculated, that the difference between the groups is basically the same as the correlation within the groups. Therefore, the regression coefficients obtained from a linear mixed model analysis are exactly the same as the regression coefficients obtained from a comparable GEE analysis. In this respect, 'comparable' means a mixed model analysis with only a random intercept and a GEE analysis with an exchangeable correlation structure are comparable. In both analyses the dependency of the observations within the groups is modelled by only one coefficient, either the difference between the groups or the correlation within the groups.

However, when the result of a logistic mixed model analysis is compared to the result of a logistic GEE analysis, the results are not the same. This is caused by another difference between mixed model analysis and GEE analysis. Basically, separate regression coefficients are calculated for the different groups in both methods, after which the overall regression coefficient is obtained by either taking the average of the group regression coefficients (GEE analysis) or the median of the group regression coefficients (mixed model analysis). GEE analysis is therefore also known as a population average approach, while mixed model analysis is also known as a group-specific approach. In regard to the results of a linear regression analysis it does not make a difference, but in regard to the results of a logistic regression analysis, it does. In fact, the regression coefficients obtained from a logistic mixed model analysis will always be higher compared to the regression coefficients obtained from a logistic GEE analysis.

This difference is based on a mathematical relationship (see Eq. 4.2) and depends on the magnitude of the between-group variance (Ten Have et al., 2004; Heo and Leon, 2005). When there is more between-group variance, the difference between the regression coefficients will be larger.

$$\beta^{(\text{GEE})} = \left[\left(\frac{16\sqrt{3}}{15\pi} \right)^2 \sigma_b^2 + 1 \right]^{-1/2} \beta^{(\text{mixed})} \tag{4.2a}$$

$$\frac{16\sqrt{3}}{15\pi} = 0.588 \tag{4.2b}$$

where $\beta^{(\text{GEE})}$ is the regression coefficient obtained from a logistic GEE analysis, σ_b^2 is between-group variance, $\pi = 3.14$ and $\beta^{(\text{mixed})}$ is the regression coefficient obtained from a logistic mixed model analysis.

4.5.1 Example

To illustrate the difference between a logistic mixed model analysis and a logistic GEE analysis, the relationship between physical activity and the dichotomous health indicator was analysed with a logistic GEE analysis as well. Output 4.6 shows the result of the logistic GEE analysis (with an exchangeable correlation structure) to analyse this relationship.

Output 4.6 Result of a logistic GEE analysis of the relationship between physical activity and the dichotomous health indicator with an exchangeable correlation structure

```
GEE population-averaged model              Number of obs      =       684
Group variable:            neighbourh~d    Number of groups   =        48
Link:                             logit    Obs per group:
Family:                        binomial                  min =         4
Correlation:              exchangeable                   avg =      14.3
                                                         max =        49
                                           Wald chi2(1)       =     75.56
Scale parameter:                      1    Prob > chi2        =    0.0000

                  (Std. Err. adjusted for clustering on neighbourhood)
-----------------------------------------------------------------------
             |              Robust
 health_dich |     Coef.   Std. Err.      z    P>|z|    [95% Conf. Interval]
-------------+---------------------------------------------------------
    activity |   .154026   .0177195     8.69   0.000     .1192964    .1887555
       _cons | -7.561609   .9067116    -8.34   0.000    -9.338731   -5.784487
-----------------------------------------------------------------------
```

When the result of the logistic GEE analysis is compared to the result of the logistic mixed model analysis, it can be seen that the regression coefficient obtained from the logistic GEE analysis is slightly lower that the regression coefficient obtained from the logistic mixed model analysis (0.15 versus 0.17). Based on Eq. 4.2 and the between-group variance estimated with the logistic mixed model analysis, this difference was as expected. Although the difference between the two regression coefficients is not very big due to the relatively low between-group variance, it is important to figure out which of the two methods provides the most valid results. Therefore, another example was performed in which the dataset used in Chapter 3 was used. The continuous outcome variable health was dichotomised by the median, and this dichotomous outcome was used to estimate the effect of the intervention. Due to ties, the dichotomisation led to observed frequencies of 43% (bad health) and 57% (good health). As has been mentioned in Chapter 3, the intervention was performed by 20 GPs, so the analysis must be adjusted for GP by using either a logistic mixed model analysis or a logistic GEE analysis. Output 4.7 shows the result of the logistic mixed model analysis with only a random intercept and Output 4.8 shows the results of the logistic GEE analysis with an exchangeable correlation structure to estimate the intervention effect.

Output 4.7 Result of a logistic mixed model analysis performed to determine the effect of the intervention on a dichotomous health outcome with a random intercept on GP level

```
Mixed-effects logistic regression            Number of obs    =        200
Group variable:             gp               Number of groups =         20

                                             Obs per group:
                                                          min =         10
                                                          avg =       10.0
                                                          max =         10

Integration method: mvaghermite              Integration pts. =          7

                                             Wald chi2(1)     =       4.74
Log likelihood = -127.58147                  Prob > chi2      =     0.0295
-------------------------------------------------------------------------------
 health_dich |     Coef.   Std. Err.      z    P>|z|     [95% Conf. Interval]
-------------+-----------------------------------------------------------------
intervention |  .7007323   .3219256     2.18   0.030     .0697698    1.331695
       _cons | -.3360448   .3342991    -1.01   0.315    -.9912589    .3191694
-------------+-----------------------------------------------------------------
gp           |
    var(_cons)|  1.195161   .6344354                      .4222577    3.382794
-------------------------------------------------------------------------------
LR test vs. logistic model: chibar2(01) = 18.16      Prob >= chibar2 = 0.0000
```

Output 4.8 Result of a logistic GEE analysis performed to determine the effect of the intervention on a dichotomous health outcome with an exchangeable correlation structure

```
GEE population-averaged model              Number of obs     =        200
Group variable:                      gp    Number of groups  =         20
Link:                             logit    Obs per group:
Family:                        binomial                        min =        10
Correlation:              exchangeable                          avg =      10.0
                                                                max =        10
                                           Wald chi2(1)       =       3.01
Scale parameter:                      1    Prob > chi2        =     0.0826

                                   (Std. Err. adjusted for clustering on gp)
------------------------------------------------------------------------------
             |               Robust
 health_dich |     Coef.    Std. Err.      z    P>|z|     [95% Conf. Interval]
-------------+----------------------------------------------------------------
intervention |   .5637023   .3247829     1.74   0.083    -.0728604    1.200265
       _cons |  -.2818512   .2665571    -1.06   0.290    -.8042935     .2405912
------------------------------------------------------------------------------
```

From Output 4.7 and Output 4.8 it can be seen that the regression coefficient obtained from the logistic mixed model analysis is much higher than the regression coefficient obtained from the logistic GEE analysis. The difference between the two regression coefficients is bigger than the difference observed in the earlier example, in which we investigated the relationship between physical activity and a dichotomous health indicator. This is caused by the relatively high between-group variance (1.195) in the second example. To evaluate which of the two methods provides the most valid results, the predicted probabilities from the two methods were compared with the observed frequencies in the data. The predicted probabilities from a logistic regression analysis can be calculated with the following equation (Eq. 4.3);

$$P(y = 1) = \frac{1}{1 + \text{EXP}\left(-\beta_0 + \beta_1 x\right)} \tag{4.3}$$

When the predicted probability is calculated with the regression coefficients of both regression equations, the predicted probability for a good health in the intervention group is 0.59 for the logistic mixed model analysis and 0.57 for the logistic GEE analysis. It was already mentioned that the observed percentage of subjects with good health in the intervention group equals 57%. In other words, with the logistic GEE analysis the predicted probability is exactly the same as the observed percentage, while the predicted probability based on the results of the logistic mixed model analysis overestimates the observed probability. Based on this simple comparison, it can be concluded that the logistic GEE analysis leads to more valid results than the logistic mixed model analysis and should therefore be preferred. For more examples showing the difference between logistic mixed model analysis and logistic GEE analysis, reference is made to Twisk et al. (2017).

One of the limitations of a (logistic) GEE analysis is that it is not possible to take into account clustering on more than one level. So, for instance, when GPs are also clustered within institutes, that correlation cannot be taken into account. When the number of institutes is relatively small, this variable could be added as a covariate (represented by dummy variables) to the model. It has been mentioned before that when the number of groups is relatively high this is, however, not really a good option. Mixed model analysis is capable of dealing with clustering on more than one level. So, when the clustering on the third level also must be taken into account in the analysis with a dichotomous outcome, a logistic mixed model analysis should be used, which leads to the same problems as has been shown before in this chapter.

The simplest solution to this problem is to ignore the clustering on the third level and to use a logistic GEE analysis only taking into account the correlated observations on the second level. The effect of this ignoring approach depends, of course, on the magnitude of the between-group variance on the third level. An alternative solution is to use a logistic mixed model analysis taking into account the clustering on both levels and to transform the obtained group-specific regression coefficient into a population average regression coefficient by using Eq. 4.2. However, in the latter the estimated regression coefficient will still highly depend on the estimation procedure used in the logistic mixed model analysis (see also Section 13.4.3).

Mixed Model Analysis with Different Outcome Variables

5.1 Introduction

In the foregoing chapters, mixed model analysis was explained with examples from studies with a continuous outcome variable (i.e. linear mixed model analysis) and a dichotomous outcome variable (i.e. logistic mixed model analysis). One of the biggest advantages of mixed model analysis is that it can be used for the analysis of other kinds of outcome variables as well. Multinomial logistic mixed model analysis can be used for categorical outcome variables and Poisson mixed model analysis or negative binomial mixed model analysis can be used for count outcome variables. Furthermore, it is possible to perform a survival mixed model analysis, although the necessary software has not yet been fully developed for this type of analysis. Again, the basic principles of all mixed model analyses are the same, meaning that all mixed model analyses are extensions of the comparable regression analysis in which an additional adjustment can be made for categorical variables with many groups. This is done by estimating the variance of the intercepts (i.e. random intercept) and/or by estimating the variance of the regression coefficients of independent variables (i.e. random slopes). As always, the necessity of the additional random intercept and/or random slopes can be evaluated with the likelihood ratio test.

5.2 Categorical Outcome Variables

When the outcome variable is categorical, multinomial logistic mixed model analysis can be applied. As for all other mixed model analyses, multinomial logistic mixed model analysis is an extension of standard multinomial logistic regression analysis. For those who are not familiar with multinomial logistic regression analysis: a multinomial logistic regression analysis is basically a sort of mixture of logistic regression analyses, in which the different categories are compared to a reference category. Therefore, as a result of multinomial logistic regression analysis, different odds ratios are obtained. When a mixed model data structure exists, a mixed model extension can also be applied for multinomial logistic regression analysis.

5.2.1 Example

In the example dataset, the outcome variable health (which was used as a continuous outcome in Chapter 2 and as a dichotomous outcome in Chapter 4) is divided into three groups: a group of patients with relatively bad heath, a group of patients with relatively moderate health and a group of patients with relatively good health. In the example dataset regarding the outcome variable, the population is almost equally divided among the three health groups (see Table 5.1). Again, the research question of interest is the relationship between physical activity and health, with the subjects living in 48 neighbourhoods. Table 5.1 shows descriptive information of the dataset used in this example.

Output 5.1 shows the result of the multinomial logistic mixed model analysis to analyse the relationship between physical activity and the categorical health indicator with a random intercept on neighbourhood level.

Output 5.1 looks slightly different from the outputs shown so far in the other chapters. This has to do with the fact that the multinomial logistic mixed model analysis was performed with a different procedure in STATA. This procedure is called 'generalised linear latent and mixed models' (gllamm) (for details, see Rabe-Hesketh and Pickles, 1999; Rabe-Hesketh et al., 2000; Rabe-Hesketh et al., 2004; Zheng and Rabe-Hesketh, 2007).

Table 5.1 Descriptive information regarding the example dataset

	Mean	Standard deviation
Physical activity	50.2	5.8
	Percentage	
Health (bad/moderate/good)	33.9% / 30.3% / 35.8%	

Output 5.1 Result of a multinomial logistic mixed model analysis of the relationship between physical activity and the categorical health indicator with a random intercept on neighbourhood level

```
gllamm model

log likelihood = -661.70299
```

health_cat	Coef.	Std. Err.	z	P>|z|	[95% Conf. Interval]
c1					
activity	.144349	.0222215	6.50	0.000	.1007957 .1879024
_cons	-7.104705	1.147547	-6.19	0.000	-9.353856 -4.855555
c2					
activity	.248994	.0243622	10.22	0.000	.2012448 .2967431
_cons	-12.34848	1.280975	-9.64	0.000	-14.85914 -9.837812

```
Variances and covariances of random effects
------------------------------------------------------------------------
***level 2 (neighbourhood)

    var(1): .8983915 (.3159563)
------------------------------------------------------------------------
```

In the earlier outputs, the last line of the output showed the result of a likelihood ratio test comparing the particular model with a naive model without any random coefficients. Because this is not the case for the gllamm procedure, the $-2 \log$ likelihood of the multinomial logistic mixed model analysis with a random intercept ($-2 \times -661.70299 = 1323.4$) must be compared with the $-2 \log$ likelihood of the multinomial logistic mixed model without a random intercept. Output 5.2 shows the result of the naive multinomial logistic regression analysis.

From Output 5.2 it can be seen that the $-2 \log$ likelihood of the naive model equals 1357.9 (-2×-678.97335). The difference between the $-2 \log$ likelihoods equals 34.5, which is highly significant on a Chi-square distribution with one degree of freedom. So, in this example, a random intercept on neighbourhood level is necessary.

For a better interpretation of the regression coefficients, Output 5.3 shows the result of the same analysis in which the regression coefficients are transformed into odds ratios.

The first odds ratio ($\exp(b)$) shown in Output 5.3 indicates that the odds ratio for a one unit difference in physical activity to be in the moderate health category compared to be in the bad health category is 1.16. The second odds ratio indicates that the odds ratio for a one unit difference in

Output 5.2 Result of a (naive) multinomial logistic regression analysis of the relationship between physical activity and the categorical health indicator

```
Multinomial logistic regression                    Number of obs   =      684
                                                   LR chi2(2)      =   141.65
                                                   Prob > chi2     =   0.0000
Log likelihood = -678.97335                        Pseudo R2       =   0.0945

-------------------------------------------------------------------------------
  health_cat |     Coef.   Std. Err.      z    P>|z|     [95% Conf. Interval]
-------------+-----------------------------------------------------------------
bad          |  (base outcome)
-------------+-----------------------------------------------------------------
moderate     |
    activity |  .1157519   .0189588    6.11   0.000     .0785933    .1529105
       _cons | -5.75327    .9316344   -6.18   0.000.   -7.57924    -3.9273
-------------+-----------------------------------------------------------------
good         |
    activity |  .218902    .0211331   10.36   0.000     .1774818    .2603221
       _cons | -10.91996  1.067365   -10.23   0.000    -13.01196   -8.827966
-------------------------------------------------------------------------------
```

Output 5.3 Result of a multinomial logistic mixed model analysis of the relationship between physical activity and the categorical health indicator with a random intercept on neighbourhood level with the effect estimates expressed as odds ratios

```
gllamm model

log likelihood = -661.70299

-------------------------------------------------------------------------------
  health_cat |    exp(b)   Std. Err.      z    P>|z|     [95% Conf. Interval]
-------------+-----------------------------------------------------------------
c1           |
    activity |  1.155287   .0256722    6.50   0.000     1.106051    1.206716
       _cons |  .0008212   .0009424   -6.19   0.000     .0000866    .007785
-------------+-----------------------------------------------------------------
c2           |
    activity |  1.282734   .0312503   10.22   0.000     1.222924    1.34547
       _cons |  4.34e-06   5.55e-06   -9.64   0.000     3.52e-07    .0000534
-------------------------------------------------------------------------------


Variances and covariances of random effects
-------------------------------------------------------------------------------

***level 2 (neighbourhood)

    var(1): .8983915 (.3159563)
-------------------------------------------------------------------------------
```

physical activity to be in the good health category compared to be in the bad health category is 1.28. So, in the multinomial logistic mixed model analysis, two mixed model logistic regression analyses are performed at the same time.

Output 5.4 Result of a multinomial logistic mixed model analysis of the relationship between physical activity and the categorical health indicator with a random intercept and a random slope for activity on neighbourhood level

```
gllamm model

log likelihood = -660.81751
```

health_cat	Coef.	Std. Err.	z	P>|z|	[95% Conf. Interval]	
c1						
activity	.1474771	.0226355	6.52	0.000	.1031123	.191842
_cons	-7.2186	1.110743	-6.50	0.000	-9.395616	-5.041584
c2						
activity	.252497	.024657	10.24	0.000	.2041702	.3008238
_cons	-12.48174	1.234305	-10.11	0.000	-14.90094	-10.06255

```
Variances and covariances of random effects
----------------------------------------------------------------

***level 2 (neighbourhood)

    var(1): 1.2985489 (5.0186377)
    cov(1,2): -.00949982 (.07074015)  cor(1,2): -.47472237

    var(2): .00030838 (.00087659)
----------------------------------------------------------------
```

The next step in the modelling strategy is to add a random slope for activity to the model. Output 5.4 shows the result of that analysis.

Looking at the $-2\log$ likelihood of the model with both a random intercept and a random slope for activity (Output 5.4), it can be seen that the difference between the two $-2\log$ likelihoods is very small ($-2 \times -660.81751 = 1321.6$ versus 1323.4) and not statistically significant on a Chi-square distribution with two degrees of freedom. There are two degrees of freedom because, besides the random slope variance, the covariance between the random intercept and random slope is also added to the model. Therefore, the model with only a random intercept is preferable.

In the present example the categorical outcome variable is basically an ordinal variable, and it is sometimes suggested that in such a situation an ordered multinomial logistic mixed model analysis should be performed. In the present example, the multinomial logistic mixed model analysis resulted in two regression coefficients. In an ordered multinomial logistic mixed model analysis, one regression coefficient is estimated. This regression

Output 5.5 Result of an ordered multinomial logistic mixed model analysis of the relationship between physical activity and the categorical health indicator with a random intercept on neighbourhood level

```
Mixed-effects ologit regression              Number of obs     =        684
Group variable:   neighbourhood              Number of groups  =         48

                                             Obs per group:
                                                          min =          4
                                                          avg =       14.3
                                                          max =         49

Integration method: mvaghermite              Integration pts.  =          7

                                             Wald chi2(1)      =     121.51
Log likelihood = -659.34999                  Prob > chi2       =     0.0000
-------------+---------------------------------------------------------------
  health_cat |     Coef.   Std. Err.      z    P>|z|     [95% Conf. Interval]
-------------+---------------------------------------------------------------
    activity |   .1822405   .0165324    11.02   0.000     .1498376    .2146434
-------------+---------------------------------------------------------------
       /cut1 |   8.312485   .8314028    10.00   0.000     6.682965    9.942004
       /cut2 |   9.951651   .8622305    11.54   0.000      8.26171   11.64159
-------------+---------------------------------------------------------------
neighbourh~d |
   var(_cons)|   .5693115   .1971979                       .2887428   1.122506
-----------------------------------------------------------------------------
LR test vs. ologit model: chibar2(01) = 36.19        Prob >= chibar2 = 0.0000
```

coefficient accounts for the difference between the moderate health category and the bad health category, but also for the difference between the good health category and the moderate health category. With this method the ordinal nature of the outcome variable is taken into account, assuming the steps between the different categories are equal. Output 5.5 shows the result of the ordered multinomial logistic mixed model analysis in order to analyse the relationship between physical activity and the categorical health indicator with a random intercept on neighbourhood level. For the ordered multinomial logistic mixed model analysis, there is a general procedure available (meologit) in STATA, so there is no need to use the gllamm procedure.

From the last line in Output 5.5 it can be seen that a model with a random intercept is significantly better than a model without a random intercept. The difference in -2 log likelihood between a model with a random intercept and a model without a random intercept is 36.19, and, evaluated on a Chi-square distribution with one degree of freedom, this is highly significant. Thus, a random intercept is necessary in this analysis. Looking at the fixed part of the model, it can be seen that there is one regression coefficient for activity. This coefficient accounts for the

Output 5.6 Result of an ordered logistic mixed model analysis of the relationship between physical activity (centred) and the categorical health indicator with a random intercept and a random slope for activity on neighbourhood level

```
Mixed-effects ologit regression              Number of obs     =        684
Group variable:   neighbourhood              Number of groups  =         48

                                             Obs per group:
                                                          min =          4
                                                          avg =       14.3
                                                          max =         49

Integration method: mvaghermite              Integration pts.  =          7

                                             Wald chi2(1)      =      81.15
Log likelihood = -658.16488                  Prob > chi2       =     0.0000
-------------------------------------------------------------------------------
  health_cat |     Coef.   Std. Err.      z    P>|z|    [95% Conf. Interval]
-------------+-----------------------------------------------------------------
 activity_c~t |  .1920165   .0213155    9.01   0.000    .1502389    .2337941
-------------+-----------------------------------------------------------------
       /cut1 | -.8285672    .152158    -5.45   0.000   -1.126791   -.530343
       /cut2 |  .8373246   .1536077     5.45   0.000    .5362591    1.13839
-------------+-----------------------------------------------------------------
neighbourh~d |
var(activi~t)|  .0044098    .003831               .0008034    .0242044
  var(_cons) |  .5920081    .211181               .2942302    1.191155
-------------+-----------------------------------------------------------------
neighbourh~d |
  cov(_cons, |
activity_c~t)| -.0069235     .02024    -0.34   0.732   -.0465932    .0327461
-------------------------------------------------------------------------------
LR test vs. ologit model: chi2(3) = 38.56            Prob > chi2 = 0.0000
```

difference in outcome between moderate health and bad health and between good health and moderate health. It should be noted that the obtained regression coefficient is a sort of average of the two regression coefficients obtained from the multinomial logistic mixed model analysis, the result of which was shown in Output 5.3.

The next step in the analysis is to add a random slope for activity to the model. To obtain a valid result of this analysis, it was necessary to centre the independent variable physical activity (see Sections 2.5 and 2.6.1). Output 5.6 shows the result of this analysis.

From Output 5.6 it can be seen that a random slope for activity is not necessary. The difference between the -2 log likelihood of a model without a random slope ($-2 \times -659.34999 = 1318.7$) and the -2 log likelihood of a model with a random slope ($-2 \times -658.16488 = 1316.3$) is 2.4, which, evaluated on a Chi-square distribution with two degrees of freedom is not statistically significant. So, regarding the ordered multinomial logistic regression analysis, a model with only a random intercept is preferable too.

Although the ordered multinomial logistic mixed model analysis is more efficient than the standard multinomial logistic mixed model analysis, because fewer regression coefficients are estimated, it is questionable whether the assumption of the ordered multinomial mixed model analysis holds in many situations. It is maybe better to perform a standard multinomial logistic mixed model analysis, especially when the number of categories is relatively small.

5.3 Count Outcome Variables

A special case of a categorical outcome variable is a count variable. Because count outcome variables, such as the number of physical complaints, the number of epileptic seizures, the number of asthma attacks, etc. normally have a Poisson distribution, Poisson regression analysis is mostly used to analyse count outcome variables. A Poisson distribution is characterised by a discrete variable which is skewed to the right and where the mean value is more or less equal to the variance. For a Poisson regression analysis, a mixed model extension is also available to take into account clustering of the data, i.e. to adjust for a categorical variable with many categories. The basic principle behind a Poisson mixed model analysis is the same as for all other mixed model analyses: by adding a random intercept to the model, an adjustment is made for the particular categorical variable, and by adding a random slope to the model, the regression coefficient for a particular variable is assumed to be different for the different groups.

5.3.1 Example

The example dataset consists of 518 elderly people living in 12 nursing homes. The outcome variable is the number of falls and the research aim of interest is the relationship between age and the number of falls. Table 5.2 shows the descriptive information of the example dataset.

From Table 5.2 it can be seen that the outcome variable (the number of falls) is more or less Poisson distributed, although the variance is slightly higher than the mean value. Output 5.7 shows the result of the Poisson mixed model analysis to analyse the relationship between age and the number of falls. The model includes a random intercept on nursing home level to take into account the correlated observations within the nursing homes.

First of all, it can be seen from Output 5.7 that it is necessary to add a random intercept to the model. The last line of the output shows the result of the likelihood ratio test, in which the model with a random intercept is compared to a naive Poisson regression model without an adjustment for nursing home. The p-value of the likelihood ratio is 0.0008, which is highly significant.

Table 5.2 Descriptive information regarding the example dataset

	Mean	Standard deviation
Age	82.7	7.7
Number of falls	0.76	1.01
	Number	Percentage
Number of falls		
0	271	52.5%
1	152	29.3%
2	52	10.1%
3	30	5.8%
4	12	2.3%

Output 5.7 Result of a Poisson mixed model analysis of the relationship between age and the number of falls with a random intercept on nursing home level

```
Mixed-effects Poisson regression          Number of obs    =        518
Group variable:            home           Number of groups =         12

                                          Obs per group:
                                                        min =         27
                                                        avg =       43.2
                                                        max =         58

Integration method: mvaghermite           Integration pts. =          7

                                          Wald chi2(1)     =       6.23
Log likelihood = -622.22667               Prob > chi2      =     0.0125
-------------------------------------------------------------------------
       falls |    Coef.   Std. Err.      z    P>|z|    [95% Conf. Interval]
-------------+-----------------------------------------------------------
         age |  .0173399  .0069456     2.50   0.013    .0037268    .030953
       _cons | -1.746404  .5876569    -2.97   0.003   -2.89819   -.5946173
-------------+-----------------------------------------------------------
home         |
   var(_cons)|  .0592785  .0381132                     .0168119   .2090155
-------------------------------------------------------------------------
LR test vs. Poisson model: chibar2(01) = 10.07      Prob >= chibar2 = 0.0008
```

In the fixed part of the regression model it can be seen that the regression coefficient for age equals 0.0173399. This regression coefficient can be transformed into a rate ratio by taking EXP[regression coefficient]. It is also possible to directly obtain the rate ratio in the output (see Output 5.8).

The rate ratio shown in Output 5.8 (1.017491) indicates that for each year difference in age, the number of falls by elderly people is 1.02 times as high.

In the example it was shown that the outcome variable was more or less Poisson distributed, although the variance was slightly higher than the mean value. It should be noted that in many situations the variance of the distribution of a count outcome variable is much higher than the mean value. This phenomenon is known as overdispersion, and when there is a lot of over-dispersion, the outcome variable can be better analysed with a negative binomial regression analysis. Negative binomial regression analysis is basic-ally the same as Poisson regression analysis, but it is known from the literature that negative binomial regression is preferable over Poisson regres-sion when there is overdispersion in the count outcome variable (Gardner et al., 1995; Hutchinson and Holtman, 2005; Weaver et al., 2015). Also, for a negative binomial regression analysis, a mixed model extension is available. And as for all other outcomes, negative binomial mixed model analysis is an extension of standard negative binomial regression analysis in which an

Output 5.8 Result of a Poisson mixed model analysis of the relationship between age and the number of falls with a random intercept on nursing home level with the effect estimate expressed as rate ratio

```
Mixed-effects Poisson regression              Number of obs     =       518
Group variable:           home                Number of groups  =        12

                                              Obs per group:
                                                            min =        27
                                                            avg =      43.2
                                                            max =        58

Integration method: mvaghermite               Integration pts.  =         7

                                              Wald chi2(1)      =      6.23
Log likelihood = -622.22667                   Prob > chi2       =    0.0125
-----------------------------------------------------------------------------
       falls |      IRR   Std. Err.      z    P>|z|     [95% Conf. Interval]
-------------+---------------------------------------------------------------
         age |  1.017491   .0070671    2.50   0.013     1.003734    1.031437
       _cons |     .1744   .1024874   -2.97   0.003      .0551229    .5517737
-------------+---------------------------------------------------------------
home         |
    var(_cons)|  .0592785   .0381132                      .0168119    .2090155
-----------------------------------------------------------------------------
LR test vs. Poisson model: chibar2(01) = 10.07         Prob >= chibar2 = 0.0008
```

Output 5.9 Result of a negative binomial mixed model analysis of the relationship between age and the number of falls with a random intercept on nursing home level

```
Mixed-effects nbinomial regression          Number of obs     =       518
Overdispersion:           mean
Group variable:           home              Number of groups  =        12

                                            Obs per group:
                                                          min =        27
                                                          avg =      43.2
                                                          max =        58

Integration method: mvaghermite            Integration pts.  =         7

                                            Wald chi2(1)      =      4.72
Log likelihood = -614.03272                 Prob > chi2       =    0.0298
-------------------------------------------------------------------------
      falls |     Coef.   Std. Err.      z    P>|z|   [95% Conf. Interval]
------------+------------------------------------------------------------
        age |   .0173359   .0079779    2.17   0.030    .0016996    .0329722
      _cons |  -1.74134    .6718858   -2.59   0.010   -3.058211   -.4244677
------------+------------------------------------------------------------
   /lnalpha |  -.9215672   .3143356   -2.93   0.003   -1.537654   -.3054808
------------+------------------------------------------------------------
home        |
   var(_cons)| .0507419   .0383603                     .011531     .2232882
-------------------------------------------------------------------------
LR test vs. nbinomial model: chibar2(01) = 5.02        Prob >= chibar2 = 0.0125
```

adjustment can be made for a categorical variable with many groups by adding a random intercept to the model. Output 5.9 shows the result of a negative binomial mixed model analysis to investigate the relationship between age and the number of falls, with a random intercept on nursing home level. This is the same analysis as has been performed with Poisson mixed model analysis; the result was shown in Output 5.7.

Because the outcome variable was more or less Poisson distributed, there is not much difference between the results of a Poisson mixed model analysis and a negative binomial mixed model analysis. For the negative binomial mixed model analysis, the regression coefficient can be transformed into a rate ratio, and this rate ratio can also be directly obtained from the output (see Output 5.10).

Because in the above example the amount of overdispersion was small, the result of a Poisson mixed model analysis was almost the same as the result of a negative binomial mixed model analysis. In a second example, the amount of overdispersion is much bigger (see Table 5.3). The data contains the results of an intervention study aiming to reduce the number of falls in elderly people. The intervention was performed in the same 518 subjects living in the same 12 nursing homes as in the first example.

Output 5.10 Result of a negative binomial mixed model analysis of the relationship between age and the number of falls with a random intercept on nursing home level with the effect estimate expressed as rate ratio

```
Mixed-effects nbinomial regression          Number of obs      =        518
Overdispersion:            mean             Numbèr of groups   =         12
Group variable:            home

                                            Obs per group:
                                                       min =         27
                                                       avg =       43.2
                                                       max =         58

Integration method: mvaghermite              Integration pts.  =          7

                                            Wald chi2(1)       =       4.72
Log likelihood = -614.03272                 Prob > chi2        =     0.0298
-------------------------------------------------------------------------------
      falls |       IRR    Std. Err.      z    P>|z|     [95% Conf. Interval]
------------+------------------------------------------------------------------
        age |   1.017487    .0081174    2.17   0.030     1.001701    1.033522
      _cons |   .1752854    .1177718   -2.59   0.010     .0469716    .6541179
------------+------------------------------------------------------------------
    /lnalpha |  -.9215672    .3143356   -2.93   0.003    -1.537654   -.3054808
------------+------------------------------------------------------------------
home        |
  var(_cons)|   .0507419    .0383603                      .011531    .2232882
-------------------------------------------------------------------------------
LR test vs. nbinomial model: chibar2(01) = 5.02     Prob >= chibar2 = 0.0125
```

Table 5.3 Descriptive information regarding the example dataset

	Mean	Standard deviation
Number of falls	1.5	2.7
	Percentage	
Intervention (no/yes)	52% / 48%	

From Table 5.3 it can be seen that the outcome variable, i.e. the number of falls, shows a big overdispersion. The variance ($2.7^2 = 7.29$) is much higher than the mean value (1.5). Output 5.11 shows the result of the Poisson mixed model analysis to analyse the effect of the intervention with a random intercept on nursing home level, while Output 5.12 shows the result of the negative binomial mixed model analysis.

From Output 5.11 and Output 5.12 it can be seen that the regression coefficients obtained from the two analyses are different from each other. The regression coefficient obtained from the Poisson mixed model analysis (−0.1985429) is more negative than the one obtained from the negative binomial mixed model analysis (−0.1749055), indicating a stronger effect

Output 5.11 Result of a Poisson mixed model analysis to determine the effect of the intervention on the number of falls with a random intercept on nursing home level

```
Mixed-effects Poisson regression          Number of obs      =        518
Group variable:            home           Number of groups   =         12

                                          Obs per group:
                                                        min =         27
                                                        avg =       43.2
                                                        max =         58

Integration method: mvaghermite           Integration pts.   =          7

                                          Wald chi2(1)       =       0.47
Log likelihood = -1149.5568               Prob > chi2        =     0.4932
-----------------------------------------------------------------------------
       falls |      Coef.   Std. Err.      z    P>|z|     [95% Conf. Interval]
-------------+---------------------------------------------------------------
intervention |  -.1985429   .2897549    -0.69   0.493    -.766452    .3693662
       _cons |   .3779185    .203391     1.86   0.063   -.0207206    .7765576
-------------+---------------------------------------------------------------
home         |
   var(_cons)|   .2312561   .1041141                     .0956913    .5588738
-----------------------------------------------------------------------------
LR test vs. Poisson model: chibar2(01) = 122.26      Prob >= chibar2 = 0.0000
```

Output 5.12 Result of a negative binomial mixed model analysis to determine the effect of the intervention on the number of falls with a random intercept on nursing home level

```
Mixed-effects nbinomial regression        Number of obs      =        518
Overdispersion:            mean
Group variable:            home           Number of groups   =         12

                                          Obs per group:
                                                        min =         27
                                                        avg =       43.2
                                                        max =         58

Integration method: mvaghermite           Integration pts.   =          7

                                          Wald chi2(1)       =       0.37
Log likelihood = -829.53333               Prob > chi2        =     0.5420
-----------------------------------------------------------------------------
       falls |      Coef.   Std. Err.      z    P>|z|     [95% Conf. Interval]
-------------+---------------------------------------------------------------
intervention |  -.1749055   .2868255    -0.61   0.542    -.7370731   .3872621
       _cons |    .398564    .200014     1.99   0.046     .0065437   .7905842
-------------+---------------------------------------------------------------
    /lnalpha |   .7769115   .1078742     7.20   0.000     .5654819   .9883412
-------------+---------------------------------------------------------------
home         |
   var(_cons)|   .1726614   .1025805                      .0538871   .5532302
-----------------------------------------------------------------------------
LR test vs. nbinomial model: chibar2(01) = 12.36     Prob >= chibar2 = 0.0002
```

estimated with the Poisson mixed model analysis. On top of that, the random intercept variance is higher when obtained from the Poisson mixed model analysis than when obtained from the negative binomial mixed model analysis. As has been mentioned before, when there is overdispersion, it is known from the literature that a negative binomial mixed model analysis is preferable over a Poisson mixed model analysis (Gardner et al., 1995; Hutchinson and Holtman, 2005; Weaver et al., 2015).

5.4 Survival Data

Logistic mixed model analyses were discussed in Chapter 4. Logistic mixed model analysis can be used to analyse a dichotomous outcome variable, and in the example a dichotomous health indicator was the event of interest. When the data in a study provides not only information about whether the event of interest occurs in a subject but also at what point in time it occurs, this additional information can be included in the analysis by applying survival analysis. The main statistical technique used to analyse survival data is Cox (proportional hazards) regression analysis. In Cox regression analysis both the occurrence of the event and the time when the patient was at risk for the occurrence of that event are used as the outcome variable. Because the hazard function over time is modelled in Cox regression analysis, the result of such an analysis is a hazard ratio. At present, the only software in which mixed model Cox regression analysis can be performed is implemented in the gllamm procedure in STATA (see Section 5.2 and Chapter 13). However, this procedure is far from straightforward, and it goes beyond the scope of this book to explain it in detail (for details see Rabe-Hesketh et al., 2004). One of the reasons for this complexity probably is the fact that there is no real intercept in a Cox regression model. Because the intercept of a Cox regression model can be interpreted as the baseline hazard function it changes over time.

So, what can be done when not only is survival data available in a study, but when that data is also clustered, for instance, within neighbourhoods? In STATA there is an additional option available for the standard Cox regression analysis, which provides an adjustment for clustering of observations within groups. This analysis can therefore be seen as a primitive mixed model survival analysis.

5.4.1 Example

In the example dataset, the effect of two treatments regarding recovery from low back pain is analysed in comparison to a control condition. The subjects are treated by different therapists, so the patient data is clustered

Table 5.4 Descriptive information regarding the example dataset

	Mean	Standard deviation
Follow-up time (in weeks)	39.9	19.1
Number of therapists	12	
	Percentage	
Recovery (no/yes)	61.2% / 38.8%	
Treatment		
Control	32.4%	
Treatment 1	35.2%	
Treatment 2	32.4%	

Output 5.13 Result of a naive Cox regression analysis of the effect of the two treatments for recovery from low back pain

```
Cox regression -- Breslow method for ties

No. of subjects =          441              Number of obs   =          441
No. of failures =          171
Time at risk    =        17610
                                            LR chi2(2)      =        35.19
Log likelihood  =   -904.23884             Prob > chi2     =       0.0000

------------------------------------------------------------------------------
        _t | Haz. Ratio   Std. Err.      z    P>|z|     [95% Conf. Interval]
-----------+------------------------------------------------------------------
 treatment |
treatment 1 |   2.49493    .6154215     3.71   0.000     1.538486    4.045976
treatment 2 |   3.594673    .861099     5.34   0.000     2.247788     5.74862
------------------------------------------------------------------------------
```

within therapists. The outcome variable of interest is time to recovery, and Table 5.4 shows descriptive information regarding the example.

From Table 5.4 it can be seen that the average follow-up time was about 40 weeks (the range was between 3 and 60 weeks). Ignoring the fact that the observations are clustered within the therapist, a naive Cox regression analysis can be performed, with treatment as the only independent variable. Output 5.13 shows the results of this naive Cox regression analysis.

The first part of Output 5.13 provides some general information about the analysis. It can be seen that there are 441 observations, there are 171 subjects with recovery (i.e. the prevalence of recovery was 39%), and the total follow-up period for the entire study population is 17.610 months. Furthermore, the log likelihood of the model is shown (−904.23884) and the significance of the total model (i.e. the model with only treatment compared to a model without independent variables). The effects of the two treatments can be derived from the last part of the output, which gives the two hazard ratios. For the first treatment a hazard ratio of 2.49493 was found and for the second treatment a hazard ratio of 3.5946673 was found. So, patients who are in the first treatment group have, on average over time, a 2.49 times higher probability to recover compared to patients in the control condition. Patients who are in the second treatment group have on average over time, a 3.59 times higher probability to recover compared to patients in the control group. Furthermore, it can be seen that both hazard ratios are highly significant.

To adjust for the dependency of the observations within therapists, a stratified Cox regression analysis can be performed. Output 5.14 shows the result of this analysis.

The last line of Output 5.14 shows that the analysis is *stratified by therapist*. This means that the baseline hazard functions are allowed to differ between therapists, or in other words, the intercept is allowed to differ between therapists. To evaluate whether this random intercept is necessary, the likelihood ratio test can be applied. With this test the $-2\log$ likelihood of the two models (i.e. with and without stratification for therapist) must be compared. The $-2\log$ likelihood of the model without stratification was $-2 \times -904.23884 = 1808.5$, while the $-2\log$ likelihood of the model with stratification was $-2 \times -486.95752 = 973.9$. The difference between the $-2\log$ likelihood of the two models is therefore very big

Output 5.14 Result of a stratified Cox regression analysis of the effect of the two treatments for recovery from low back pain

```
Stratified Cox regr. -- Breslow method for ties

No. of subjects =            441           Number of obs    =          441
No. of failures =            171
Time at risk    =          17610
                                           LR chi2(2)       =        21.33
Log likelihood  =      -486.95752          Prob > chi2      =       0.0000

------------------------------------------------------------------------------
        _t | Haz. Ratio   Std. Err.      z    P>|z|     [95% Conf. Interval]
-----------+------------------------------------------------------------------
 treatment |
treatment 1 |  1.593431    .4079854    1.82   0.069     .964695    2.631945
treatment 2 |  2.751998    .6794615    4.10   0.000    1.696244    4.464858
------------------------------------------------------------------------------
                                                      Stratified by therapist
```

(1808.5 − 973.9 = 834.6). This difference, however, does not follow a Chi-square distribution with one degree of freedom. This is due to the fact that the stratified Cox regression analysis is not a real mixed model analysis. In the stratified Cox regression analysis it is not the variance of the different baseline hazard functions that is estimated but all baseline hazard functions for the different therapists. So, instead of one baseline hazard function in the naive Cox regression analysis, 12 baseline hazard functions are estimated in the stratified Cox regression analysis. In other words, the difference in −2 log likelihood of the two models must be evaluated on a Chi-square distribution with 11 degrees of freedom, which is nevertheless highly significant. The influence of allowing different baseline hazard functions for the therapists is that the hazard ratio for both treatments is much lower, and for treatment 1 the adjusted hazard ratio is not statistically significant anymore.

The results presented in Output 5.14 provide the final result of this analysis, because with a stratified Cox regression analysis it is not possible to allow the regression coefficients for treatment to differ between therapists, which is to say that it is not possible to add random slopes to the model. So, the final hazard ratio for treatment 1 is 1.59, with a 95% CI ranging from 0.96 to 2.63, and the hazard ratio for treatment 2 is 2.76, with a 95% CI ranging from 1.70 to 4.46.

Because there are no assumptions about the shape of the baseline hazard function, Cox regression analysis is known as a semi-parametric survival analysis. It is also possible to perform a parametric survival analysis in which it is assumed that the baseline hazard function has a particular shape. The parametric survival analyses used most are the one assuming an exponential baseline hazard function and the one assuming a Weibull baseline hazard function. With the exponential hazard function, the hazard is assumed to be constant over time, while with the Weibull hazard function, the hazard is assumed to increase or decrease over time (see for further details Lambert and Royston, 2009; Cleves et al., 2010; Royston and Lambert, 2011).

A mixed model extension is available in STATA for these parametric survival models. So, the treatment effects can be estimated from a parametric survival model. Output 5.15 shows the result of an exponential survival

Output 5.15 Result of an exponential survival mixed model analysis to determine the effect of the two treatments for recovery from low back pain with a random intercept on therapist level

```
Mixed-effects exponential regression      Number of obs     =        441
Group variable:         therapist         Number of groups  =         12

                                          Obs per group:
                                                       min =         36
                                                       avg =       36.8
                                                       max =         39

Integration method: mvaghermite          Integration pts.  =          7

                                          Wald chi2(2)      =      24.60
Log likelihood = -917.60176              Prob > chi2       =     0.0000
--------------------------------------------------------------------------
        _t | Haz. Ratio   Std. Err.      z    P>|z|    [95% Conf. Interval]
-----------+--------------------------------------------------------------
           |
 treatment |
treatment 1 |  1.896337    .4771252     2.54  0.011     1.15811    3.105138
treatment 2 |   3.14248     .762879     4.72  0.000    1.952684    5.057234
           |
      _cons |  .0036559    .0012105   -16.95  0.000    .0019106    .0069957
-----------+--------------------------------------------------------------
therapist  |
var(_cons) |  .7250114     .397336                     .2476575    2.122454
--------------------------------------------------------------------------
LR test vs. exponential model: chibar2(01) = 57.61   Prob >= chibar2 = 0.0000
```

mixed model analysis to determine treatment effects with a random intercept on therapist level.

In the last line of Output 5.15 it can be seen that the model with a random intercept on therapist level is significantly better that the model without a random intercept. The likelihood ratio test gives a Chi-square value of 57.61, which is highly significant on a Chi-square distribution with one degree of freedom. The hazard ratios for the two treatments are slightly higher than the ones obtained from the stratified Cox regression analysis. Output 5.16 shows the result of a Weibull survival mixed model analysis to determine treatment effects with a random intercept on therapist level.

Compared to the mixed model survival analysis assuming an exponential survival function, the hazard ratios derived from a mixed model survival analysis assuming a Weibull survival function are a bit lower and a bit closer to the hazard ratios obtained from a stratified Cox regression analysis. Also, in the Weibull survival mixed model analysis, it is obvious that a random intercept on therapist level is necessary; the Chi-square value

Output 5.16 Result of a Weibull survival mixed model analysis to determine the effect of the two treatments for recovery from low back pain with a random intercept on therapist level

```
Mixed-effects Weibull regression              Number of obs    =         441
Group variable:       therapist               Number of groups =          12

                                              Obs per group:
                                                           min =          36
                                                           avg =        36.8
                                                           max =          39

Integration method: mvaghermite               Integration pts. =           7

                                              Wald chi2(2)     =       24.47
Log likelihood = -261.43274                   Prob > chi2      =      0.0000
---------------------------------------------------------------------------
        _t | Haz. Ratio  Std. Err.      z    P>|z|    [95% Conf. Interval]
-----------+---------------------------------------------------------------
 treatment |
treatment 1 |  1.651844   .4216976    1.97   0.049    1.001536    2.724403
treatment 2 |  2.994665   .7356681    4.46   0.000    1.850301    4.846788
           |
      _cons |  .0000312   .0000209  -15.52   0.000    8.41e-06    .0001156
-----------+---------------------------------------------------------------
     /ln_p | .8084344   .0656536    12.31   0.000    .6797557    .9371131
-----------+---------------------------------------------------------------
therapist  |
  var(_cons)| .7976249   .4296272                     .2775322    2.292366
---------------------------------------------------------------------------
LR test vs. Weibull model: chibar2(01) = 64.93        Prob >= chibar2 = 0.0000
```

of the likelihood ratio test equals 64.93, which is highly significant on a Chi-square distribution with one degree of freedom.

Because the parametric survival functions are analysed within a mixed model framework it is possible to add random slopes to the model. In this particular example we could add random slopes for the two treatment variables to the survival model, allowing the treatment effects to differ between therapists. Due to the low number of therapists in this example (12), a parametric survival mixed model analysis with random slopes for the two treatment variables as well as the covariances between the random intercept and the two random slopes did not converge, so the model with only a random intercept is the final model from which the hazard ratios should be derived.

In Output 5.16 the so-called ancillary parameter is also provided (the natural log of 0.8084344). This parameter (2.23) indicates the exponential increase in hazard over time. It should be noted that when this parameter equals 1, the Weibull survival function is equal to the exponential survival function.

5.5 Other Outcomes

Within STATA there are many procedures available to perform mixed model analyses for different outcomes. However, these procedures (starting with xt) are only capable to perform a mixed model analysis with a random intercept, but not with random slopes. For instance, with the xttobit procedure, a tobit mixed model analysis can be used for skewed distributions with floor or ceiling effects due to censoring. The xtintreg procedure can be used for interval mixed model analysis and the xtivreg procedure for mixed model analysis with instrumental variables. In Chapter 13, the use of the xt procedure will be further discussed.

6

Explaining Differences between Groups

6.1 Introduction

The basic principles of mixed model analysis were discussed in Chapter 2. In this discussion, mixed model analysis was used as a very efficient way to take into account a categorical variable with many groups. In that respect, the random intercept variance was not the main interest, and the categorical variable with many groups was treated as a nuisance variable that should be taken into account. In this chapter another application of the use of mixed model analysis will be discussed. In this application the main interest is in the random intercept variance. In fact, the aim of the analysis is to explain the random intercept variance or, in other words, to explain why the groups are different regarding a particular outcome variable.

In the literature there are many examples available in which this application is used. It is used, for instance, to evaluate which variables explain health differences between neighbourhoods (Schüle et al., 2016), which variables are responsible for difference in performance between hospitals (Ghith et al., 2016), etc.

The analysis aiming to explain the random intercept variance starts with a model with only an intercept and the random variation around the intercept. Then, step by step, each of the possible explanatory variables is added to the model and the influence of the particular variables is evaluated by the amount of the random intercept variance that is explained by the particular variable. After evaluating all the possible explanatory variables, the variable which explains most of the variance is added to the model and is the new starting point for the next step in the modelling procedure. This procedure is repeated until the remaining variables are not explaining a relevant part of the variance anymore. In this modelling procedure the interest is not in the regression coefficients of the explanatory variables but in the amount of the random intercept variance that is explained.

6.2 Example

In the example, the aim of the study is to explain differences in health between neighbourhoods. The example's subjects are clustered in 28 neighbourhoods and health is measured as a continuous variable which can range between 0 and 30. Table 6.1 shows descriptive information regarding the example dataset.

From Table 6.1 it can be seen that there are four potential individual explanatory variables and two neighbourhood explanatory variables.

As has been mentioned before, the starting point of the modelling is an intercept-only model with a random intercept on neighbourhood level, without any explanatory variables. Output 6.1 shows the result of that analysis.

Basically the only part of Output 6.1 which is of interest in this particular example is the random intercept variance (1.356431). This number reflects the variance in health between neighbourhoods. In the next steps of the modelling procedure, this random intercept variance will be explained by adding both individual and neighbourhood variables to the model.

Table 6.1 Descriptive information regarding the example dataset

	Mean	Standard deviation
Health	11.98	3.97
Individual variables		
	Percentage	
Gender (females/males)	39.2%/60.8%	
Ethnicity (Caucasian/non Caucasian)	46.9%/53.1%	
Education (low/high)	77.4%/22.6%	
Physical activity (low/moderate/high)	70.3%/18.9%/10.8%	
Neighbourhood variables		
Number of playgrounds (low/high)	48.4%/51.6%	
Unemployment rate (low/high)	72.6%/27.4%	

Output 6.1 Result of a linear (intercept-only) mixed model analysis to explain health differences between neighbourhoods with a random intercept on neighbourhood level

```
Mixed-effects ML regression                     Number of obs    .=        508
Group variable: neighbourhood                   Number of groups  =         28

                                                Obs per group:
                                                            min =          3
                                                            avg =       18.1
                                                            max =         59

                                                Wald chi2(0)      =          .
Log likelihood = -1407.8299                     Prob > chi2       =          .

----------------------------------------------------------------------------
     health |     Coef.   Std. Err.      z    P>|z|    [95% Conf. Interval]
------------+---------------------------------------------------------------
      _cons |   11.97488   .2897764    41.32   0.000    11.40693    12.54283
----------------------------------------------------------------------------


----------------------------------------------------------------------------
 Random-effects Parameters   |  Estimate   Std. Err.    [95% Conf. Interval]
-----------------------------+----------------------------------------------
neighbourh~d: Identity       |
                var(_cons)   |   1.356431   .5776621     .5887043   3.125346
-----------------------------+----------------------------------------------
               var(Residual) |   14.20534   .9127292    12.52448   16.11178
----------------------------------------------------------------------------
LR test vs. linear model: chibar2(01) = 26.95          Prob >= chibar2 = 0.0000
```

Based on the random intercept variance shown in Output 6.1, the ICC for health on the neighbourhood level can be calculated (see also Section 2.3). This is done by dividing the between-neighbourhood variance (1.356) by the total variance, which is calculated by summation of the between-neighbourhood variance and the within-neighbourhood variance (1.356 + 14.205). So, in this example the ICC is: 1.356/15.561 = 0.087.

The next step in the modelling procedure is to add, one by one, the possible explanatory variables to the model. Output 6.2 shows the result of the analysis in which physical activity is added to the model.

From Output 6.2 it can be seen that the random intercept variance decreases from 1.356431 to 0.7481637, which is a decrease of about 45%. This percentage can be calculated by dividing the difference between the two variances by the random intercept variance estimated without any explanatory variables ((1.356 − 0.748)/1.356 = 0.45). From Output 6.2 it can also be seen that there is a strong relationship between physical activity and health. Both activity variables (comparing moderate activity to low activity and comparing high activity to low activity) show positive regression coefficients that are highly significant. The fact that physical activity is

Output 6.2 Result of a linear mixed model analysis to explain health differences between neighbourhoods with physical activity and a random intercept on neighbourhood level

```
Mixed-effects ML regression                   Number of obs      =        508
Group variable: neighbourhood                 Number of groups   =         28

                                              Obs per group:
                                                           min =          3
                                                           avg =       18.1
                                                           max =         59

                                              Wald chi2(2)       =      63.14
Log likelihood = -1378.6752                   Prob > chi2        =     0.0000

------------------------------------------------------------------------------
     health |     Coef.    Std. Err.      z    P>|z|    [95% Conf. Interval]
------------+-----------------------------------------------------------------
_Iactivity_1 |  1.110414   .4246562     2.61   0.009    .2781035    1.942725
_Iactivity_2 |  4.281719   .5454869     7.85   0.000    3.212584    5.350853
      _cons |  11.32403    .2628835    43.08   0.000    10.80878    11.83927
------------------------------------------------------------------------------

------------------------------------------------------------------------------
  Random-effects Parameters  |   Estimate   Std. Err.     [95% Conf. Interval]
-----------------------------+------------------------------------------------
neighbourh~d: Identity       |
                 var(_cons)  |   .7481637   .4005357      .2619985    2.136458
-----------------------------+------------------------------------------------
               var(Residual) |   12.84614   .8258512      11.32532    14.57117
------------------------------------------------------------------------------
LR test vs. linear model: chibar2(01) = 11.57        Prob >= chibar2 = 0.0003
```

significantly related to health does not directly implicates that physical activity explains health differences between neighbourhoods. When physical activity is not different between the neighbourhoods, it can never explain health differences between neighbourhoods, irrespective of the strong relationship between physical activity and health. To explain health differences between neighbourhoods, the particular variable has to be related to health and has to differ between the neighbourhoods. Note that it is not necessary that the relationship with and/or the differences between neighbourhoods are statistically significant.

The next step in the modelling procedure is to repeat the analysis performed for physical activity for all other potential explanatory variables. Output 6.3 shows the analysis in which ethnicity is added to the model.

From Output 6.3 it can be seen that ethnicity explains about 5% of the variance in health between neighbourhoods $((1.356 - 1.290)/1.356 = 0.05)$. When the other two individual variables, education and gender, are added to the starting model, it can be seen that the random intercept variance increases (see Output 6.4 and Output 6.5). This is a bit strange, but not

Output 6.3 Result of a linear mixed model analysis to explain health differences between neighbourhoods with ethnicity and a random intercept on neighbourhood level

```
Mixed-effects ML regression                  Number of obs      =        508
Group variable: neighbourhood                Number of groups   =         28

                                             Obs per group:
                                                          min =          3
                                                          avg =       18.1
                                                          max =         59

                                             Wald chi2(1)       =      18.61
Log likelihood = -1398.6909                  Prob > chi2        =     0.0000

------------------------------------------------------------------------------
      health |     Coef.   Std. Err.      z    P>|z|     [95% Conf. Interval]
-------------+----------------------------------------------------------------
   ethnicity |   1.45758   .3378598     4.31   0.000     .7953866    2.119773
       _cons |  11.28494   .3254442    34.68   0.000     10.64708     11.9228
------------------------------------------------------------------------------


------------------------------------------------------------------------------
  Random-effects Parameters  |   Estimate   Std. Err.     [95% Conf. Interval]
-----------------------------+------------------------------------------------
neighbourh~d: Identity       |
                 var(_cons)  |   1.290259   .5593539      .5516499    3.017799
-----------------------------+------------------------------------------------
               var(Residual) |   13.70961   .8813913      12.08652    15.55066
------------------------------------------------------------------------------
LR test vs. linear model: chibar2(01) = 25.15        Prob >= chibar2 = 0.0000
```

Output 6.4 Result of a linear mixed model analysis to explain health differences between neighbourhoods with education and a random intercept on neighbourhood level

```
Mixed-effects ML regression                  Number of obs      =        508
Group variable: neighbourhood                Number of groups   =         28

                                             Obs per group:
                                                          min =          3
                                                          avg =       18.1
                                                          max =         59

                                             Wald chi2(1)       =       1.77
Log likelihood = -1406.963                   Prob > chi2        =     0.1840

------------------------------------------------------------------------------
      health |     Coef.   Std. Err.      z    P>|z|     [95% Conf. Interval]
-------------+----------------------------------------------------------------
   education |   .563956   .4244559     1.33   0.184    -.2679623    1.395874
       _cons |  11.82915   .3150111    37.55   0.000     11.21174    12.44656
------------------------------------------------------------------------------


------------------------------------------------------------------------------
  Random-effects Parameters  |   Estimate   Std. Err.     [95% Conf. Interval]
-----------------------------+------------------------------------------------
neighbourh~d: Identity       |
                 var(_cons)  |   1.451177    .61605       .6314959    3.334804
-----------------------------+------------------------------------------------
               var(Residual) |   14.12352   .9085615      12.45046     16.0214
------------------------------------------------------------------------------
LR test vs. linear model: chibar2(01) = 28.06        Prob >= chibar2 = 0.0000
```

Output 6.5 Result of a linear mixed model analysis to explain health differences between neighbourhoods with gender and a random intercept on neighbourhood level

```
Mixed-effects ML regression                 Number of obs      =        508
Group variable: neighbourhood               Number of groups   =         28

                                            Obs per group:
                                                         min =          3
                                                         avg =       18.1
                                                         max =         59

                                            Wald chi2(1)       =       7.57
Log likelihood = -1404.0837                 Prob > chi2        =     0.0059

------------------------------------------------------------------------------
     health |     Coef.   Std. Err.      z    P>|z|     [95% Conf. Interval]
------------+-----------------------------------------------------------------
     gender | -.9589613   .3484507    -2.75   0.006    -1.641912   -.2760105
      _cons |  12.55701   .3621074    34.68   0.000     11.8473    13.26673
------------------------------------------------------------------------------


------------------------------------------------------------------------------
  Random-effects Parameters  |   Estimate   Std. Err.     [95% Conf. Interval]
-----------------------------+------------------------------------------------
neighbourh~d: Identity       |
                 var(_cons)  |   1.429552   .6030618      .6253419    3.268003
-----------------------------+------------------------------------------------
               var(Residual) |   13.96606   .8980898      12.31224    15.84202
------------------------------------------------------------------------------
LR test vs. linear model: chibar2(01) = 28.60        Prob >= chibar2 = 0.0000
```

uncommon in this kind of analysis. The most important conclusion of these analyses is that education does not explain health differences between neighbourhoods and that gender does not explain health differences between neighbourhoods.

After adding the individual explanatory variables one by one to the model, in the next step the neighbourhood variables are added one by one to the starting model. Output 6.6 and Output 6.7 show the results of these analyses.

From Output 6.6 and Output 6.7 it can be seen that both neighbourhood variables explain part of the health differences between the neighbourhoods. For the number of playgrounds, this percentage equals 36% $((1.356 - 0.871)/1.356 = 0.36)$ and for the unemployment rate of the neighbourhood, this percentage equals 23% $((1.356 - 1.048)/1.356 = 0.23)$.

So, based on the performed analyses so far, it can be concluded that physical activity explains most of the variance in health between neighbourhoods (45%), followed by the number of playgrounds (36%), unemployment rate (23%) and ethnicity (5%).

Output 6.6 Result of a linear mixed model analysis to explain health differences between neighbourhoods with the number of playgrounds in the neighbourhood and a random intercept on neighbourhood level

```
Mixed-effects ML regression                    Number of obs     =        508
Group variable: neighbourhood                  Number of groups  =         28

                                               Obs per group:
                                                             min =          3
                                                             avg =       18.1
                                                             max =         59

                                               Wald chi2(1)      =       7.63
Log likelihood = -1404.5301                    Prob > chi2       =     0.0057

------------------------------------------------------------------------------
      health |    Coef.   Std. Err.      z    P>|z|    [95% Conf. Interval]
-------------+----------------------------------------------------------------
playing_gro~s|  1.429947   .517591     2.76   0.006    .4154873   2.444407
       _cons |  11.3832    .3347579    34.00   0.000    10.72709   12.03932
------------------------------------------------------------------------------


------------------------------------------------------------------------------
 Random-effects Parameters  |   Estimate   Std. Err.    [95% Conf. Interval]
----------------------------+-------------------------------------------------
neighbourh~d: Identity      |
                 var(_cons) |   .8705693    .44074      .3227517   2.348216
----------------------------+-------------------------------------------------
               var(Residual)|  14.20378    .9118086    12.52452   16.10818
------------------------------------------------------------------------------
LR test vs. linear model: chibar2(01) = 13.35       Prob >= chibar2 = 0.0001
```

Output 6.7 Result of a linear mixed model analysis to explain health differences between neighbourhoods with unemployment rate of the neighbourhood and a random intercept on neighbourhood level

```
Mixed-effects ML regression                    Number of obs     =        508
Group variable: neighbourhood                  Number of groups  =         28

                                               Obs per group:
                                                             min =          3
                                                             avg =       18.1
                                                             max =         59

                                               Wald chi2(1)      =       4.92
Log likelihood = -1405.5505                    Prob > chi2       =     0.0265

------------------------------------------------------------------------------
      health |    Coef.   Std. Err.      z    P>|z|    [95% Conf. Interval]
-------------+----------------------------------------------------------------
unemployment |  1.197418   .539825     2.22   0.027    .1393808   2.255456
       _cons |  11.44234   .3613138    31.67   0.000    10.73418   12.1505
------------------------------------------------------------------------------


------------------------------------------------------------------------------
 Random-effects Parameters  |   Estimate   Std. Err.    [95% Conf. Interval]
----------------------------+-------------------------------------------------
neighbourh~d: Identity      |
                 var(_cons) |  1.047711    .4806382     .426336   2.574725
----------------------------+-------------------------------------------------
               var(Residual)|  14.18819    .9102884    12.51168   16.08936
------------------------------------------------------------------------------
LR test vs. linear model: chibar2(01) = 19.92       Prob >= chibar2 = 0.0000
```

A new starting model is used in the next modelling phase, which includes the variable that explains most of the variance, which in this example is physical activity. The three variables that explained some of the variance in health between the neighbourhoods are now added one by one to the new starting model. From those analyses, again, the percentage of explained variance in the health differences between the neighbourhoods by the other variables is calculated. Note that the amount of variance to be explained now equals 0.748 (see Output 6.2). Output 6.8, Output 6.9 and Output 6.10 show the results of these analyses.

Based on Output 6.8, Output 6.9 and Output 6.10 the percentage of additional variance in neighbourhood health explained by the three variables can be calculated. For ethnicity this percentage equals around 12% ((0.748 − 0.655)/0.748 = 0.12). For the number of playgrounds in the neighbourhood, this percentage equals around 36% ((0.748 − 0.477)/0.748 = 0.36), and for unemployment rate in the neighbourhood this percentage equals around 34% ((0.748 − 0.496)/0.748 = 0.34). So, the next best explanatory variable in this example is the number of playgrounds in

Output 6.8 Result of a linear mixed model analysis to explain health differences between neighbourhoods with physical activity and ethnicity and a random intercept on neighbourhood level

```
Mixed-effects ML regression                    Number of obs    =        508
Group variable: neighbourhood                  Number of groups =         28

                                               Obs per group:
                                                          min =          3
                                                          avg =       18.1
                                                          max =         59

                                               Wald chi2(3)     =      86.69
Log likelihood = -1368.6518                    Prob > chi2      =     0.0000

-------------------------------------------------------------------------------
     health |     Coef.    Std. Err.      z     P>|z|     [95% Conf. Interval]
------------+------------------------------------------------------------------
 Iactivity_1|   1.152449    .4163605    2.77    0.006     .3363971     1.9685
 Iactivity_2|   4.263141    .5344589    7.98    0.000     3.21562    5.310661
    ethnicity|  1.444954    .3193012    4.53    0.000     .8191356   2.070773
       _cons |  10.63237    .2952513   36.01    0.000    10.05369    11.21105
-------------------------------------------------------------------------------


-------------------------------------------------------------------------------
  Random-effects Parameters  |   Estimate   Std. Err.     [95% Conf. Interval]
-----------------------------+-------------------------------------------------
neighbourh~d: Identity       |
                 var(_cons)  |   .6548962   .3735792      .2140981    2.003236
-----------------------------+-------------------------------------------------
               var(Residual) |  12.37884   .7963995      10.91233    14.04244
-------------------------------------------------------------------------------
LR test vs. linear model: chibar2(01) = 9.41        Prob >= chibar2 = 0.0011
```

Output 6.9 Result of a linear mixed model analysis to explain health differences between neighbourhoods with physical activity and the number of playgrounds in the neighbourhood and a random intercept on neighbourhood level

```
Mixed-effects ML regression                      Number of obs    =        508
Group variable: neighbourhood                    Number of groups =         28

                                                 Obs per group:
                                                             min =          3
                                                             avg =       18.1
                                                             max =         59

                                                 Wald chi2(3)     =      72.65
Log likelihood = -1375.8777                      Prob > chi2      =     0.0000

-------------------------------------------------------------------------------
     health |     Coef.   Std. Err.      z    P>|z|     [95% Conf. Interval]
------------+------------------------------------------------------------------
_Iactivity_1 |   1.13446    .421786     2.69   0.007     .3077747    1.961145
_Iactivity_2 |  4.200435   .5434428     7.73   0.000     3.135307    5.265564
playing_gro~s|  1.095593    .438904     2.50   0.013     .2353567    1.955829
       _cons |  10.86192   .3013039    36.05   0.000     10.27138    11.45247
-------------------------------------------------------------------------------


-------------------------------------------------------------------------------
 Random-effects Parameters  |   Estimate   Std. Err.     [95% Conf. Interval]
----------------------------+--------------------------------------------------
neighbourh~d: Identity      |
                var(_cons)  |   .4769993   .3125673      .1320516    1.723026
----------------------------+--------------------------------------------------
              var(Residual) |   12.83679   .8237142      11.31974    14.55716
-------------------------------------------------------------------------------
LR test vs. linear model: chibar2(01) = 5.81           Prob >= chibar2 = 0.0080
```

the neighbourhood. Both variables together (i.e. physical activity and the number of playgrounds in the neighbourhood) explain around 65% ((1.356 − 0.477)/1.356) of the neighbourhood differences in health.

Using the model with physical activity and the number of playgrounds in the neighbourhood as explanatory variables as a new starting model, in the next step it can be investigated whether the other two variables (i.e. ethnicity and unemployment rate) explain some of the remaining differences in health between the neighbourhoods. Output 6.11 and Output 6.12 show the results of these two analyses.

Based on Output 6.11 and Output 6.12, it can be calculated how much of the remaining variance in health between the neighbourhoods is explained by ethnicity and unemployment rate of the neighbourhood. For ethnicity this percentage equals around 15% ((0.477 − 0.406)/0.477 = 0.15), while for unemployment rate in the neighbourhood, this percentage equals around 35% ((0.477 − 0.312)/0.477 = 0.35). Both variables still explain a reasonable amount of the differences in health between the neighbourhoods.

Output 6.10 Result of a linear mixed model analysis to explain health differences between neighbourhoods with physical activity and unemployment rate in the neighbourhood and a random intercept on neighbourhood level

```
Mixed-effects ML regression                    Number of obs    =        508
Group variable: neighbourhood                  Number of groups =         28

                                               Obs per group:
                                                             min =          3
                                                             avg =       18.1
                                                             max =         59

                                               Wald chi2(3)     =      71.96
Log likelihood = -1376.0316                    Prob > chi2      =     0.0000

------------------------------------------------------------------------------
      health |     Coef.   Std. Err.      z    P>|z|    [95% Conf. Interval]
-------------+----------------------------------------------------------------
  _Iactivity_1 | 1.135253   .4219788     2.69   0.007    .3081902    1.962317
  _Iactivity_2 | 4.286769   .5410982     7.92   0.000    3.226236    5.347301
  unemployment | 1.058436   .4386033     2.41   0.016     .198789    1.918082
        _cons | 10.85394   .3086651    35.16   0.000    10.24896    11.45891
------------------------------------------------------------------------------

------------------------------------------------------------------------------
  Random-effects Parameters   |   Estimate   Std. Err.    [95% Conf. Interval]
-----------------------------+------------------------------------------------
neighbourh~d: Identity       |
                 var(_cons)  |   .4962182   .3162202     .1423101    1.730253
-----------------------------+------------------------------------------------
                var(Residual)|   12.83417   .8233733     11.31772     14.5538
------------------------------------------------------------------------------
LR test vs. linear model: chibar2(01) = 6.56      Prob >= chibar2 = 0.0052
```

Output 6.11 Result of a linear mixed model analysis to explain health differences between neighbourhoods with physical activity, the number of playgrounds in the neighbourhood and ethnicity and a random intercept on neighbourhood level

```
Mixed-effects ML regression                    Number of obs    =        508
Group variable: neighbourhood                  Number of groups =         28

                                               Obs per group:
                                                             min =          3
                                                             avg =       18.1
                                                             max =         59

                                               Wald chi2(4)     =      97.71
Log likelihood = -1365.6299                    Prob > chi2      =     0.0000

------------------------------------------------------------------------------
      health |     Coef.   Std. Err.      z    P>|z|    [95% Conf. Interval]
-------------+----------------------------------------------------------------
  _Iactivity_1 | 1.173913    .413232     2.84   0.004    .3639933    1.983833
  _Iactivity_2 | 4.181149   .5321569     7.86   0.000    3.138141    5.224157
 playing_gro~s | 1.084332   .4199898     2.58   0.010    .2611676    1.907497
      ethnicity | 1.453528   .3175752     4.58   0.000    .8310919    2.075964
          _cons | 10.16952   .3261267    31.18   0.000    9.530325    10.80872
------------------------------------------------------------------------------

------------------------------------------------------------------------------
  Random-effects Parameters   |   Estimate   Std. Err.    [95% Conf. Interval]
-----------------------------+------------------------------------------------
neighbourh~d: Identity       |
                 var(_cons)  |   .4061113   .2877472      .101282    1.628387
-----------------------------+------------------------------------------------
                var(Residual)|   12.35874   .7931949     10.89792    14.01539
------------------------------------------------------------------------------
LR test vs. linear model: chibar2(01) = 4.57      Prob >= chibar2 = 0.0163
```

Output 6.12 Result of a linear mixed model analysis to explain health differences between neighbourhoods with physical activity, the number of playgrounds in the neighbourhood and unemployment rate in the neighbourhood and a random intercept on neighbourhood level

```
Mixed-effects ML regression                    Number of obs    =      508
Group variable: neighbourhood                  Number of groups =       28

                                               Obs per group:
                                                            min =        3
                                                            avg =     18.1
                                                            max =       59

                                               Wald chi2(4)     =    80.67
Log likelihood = -1374.1692                    Prob > chi2      =   0.0000

------------------------------------------------------------------------------
      health |    Coef.   Std. Err.     z    P>|z|    [95% Conf. Interval]
-------------+----------------------------------------------------------------
 _Iactivity_1 |  1.158141   .4196388   2.76   0.006    .3356639    1.980618
 _Iactivity_2 |  4.223398   .5399273   7.82   0.000    3.16516     5.281636
playing_gro~s |  .8636985   .4226081   2.04   0.041    .0354018    1.691995
 unemployment |  .8156535   .4196796   1.94   0.052   -.0069033    1.63821
        _cons | 10.59549    .3099529  34.18   0.000    9.987991   11.20298
------------------------------------------------------------------------------


------------------------------------------------------------------------------
 Random-effects Parameters  |  Estimate   Std. Err.     [95% Conf. Interval]
----------------------------+-------------------------------------------------
neighbourh~d: Identity      |
                var(_cons)  |  .3120913   .2634978      .0596506    1.632859
----------------------------+-------------------------------------------------
               var(Residual)|  12.8475    .8238868     11.33007    14.56816
------------------------------------------------------------------------------
LR test vs. linear model: chibar2(01) = 2.81          Prob >= chibar2 = 0.0469
```

Therefore, the unemployment rate of the neighbourhood is added to the new starting model. Only ethnicity has to be added to the new starting model in order to evaluate whether ethnicity still explains some of the differences in health between the neighbourhoods. Output 6.13 shows the result of this analysis.

From Output 6.13 it can be seen that ethnicity still explains some of the remaining variance in health between the neighbourhoods. The percentage of explained variance can be calculated in the same way as has been done before, i.e. $(0.312 - 0.253)/0.312 = 0.19$. So, 19% of the remaining variance in health between the neighbourhoods is explained by ethnicity.

The conclusion of the last mixed model analysis performed is that around 81% $((1.356 - 0.253)/1.356 = 0.81)$ of the health differences between neighbourhoods can be explained by physical activity, ethnicity, the number of playgrounds in the neighbourhood and the unemployment rate in the neighbourhood.

Output 6.13 Result of a linear mixed model analysis to explain health differences between neighbourhoods with physical activity, the number of playgrounds in the neighbourhood, unemployment rate in the neighbourhood and ethnicity and a random intercept on neighbourhood level

```
Mixed-effects ML regression                    Number of obs     =        508
Group variable: neighbourhood                  Number of groups  =         28

                                               Obs per group:
                                                            min =          3
                                                            avg =       18.1
                                                            max =         59

                                               Wald chi2(5)      =     107.04
Log likelihood = -1363.8101                    Prob > chi2       =     0.0000

------------------------------------------------------------------------------
      health |     Coef.   Std. Err.      z    P>|z|    [95% Conf. Interval]
-------------+----------------------------------------------------------------
  _Iactivity_1 |  1.195351   .4109061     2.91   0.004    .3899903    2.000713
  _Iactivity_2 |  4.210118   .5283571     7.97   0.000    3.174557    5.245679
  playing_gro~s |  .8532653   .4026305     2.12   0.034    .064124     1.642406
  unemployment |  .8013308   .4001277     2.00   0.045    .0170949    1.585567
      ethnicity |  1.456302   .3163983     4.60   0.000    .8361728    2.076431
        _cons |  9.910224    .331313    29.91   0.000    9.260862    10.55959
------------------------------------------------------------------------------

------------------------------------------------------------------------------
  Random-effects Parameters  |   Estimate   Std. Err.     [95% Conf. Interval]
-----------------------------+------------------------------------------------
neighbourh~d: Identity       |
                var(_cons)   |   .2528462   .2381381      .0399181     1.60156
-----------------------------+------------------------------------------------
              var(Residual)  |   12.36517   .7926468      10.90524    14.02054
------------------------------------------------------------------------------
LR test vs. linear model: chibar2(01) = 2.09       Prob >= chibar2 = 0.0742
```

7

Multivariable Modelling

7.1 Introduction

Until now, the explanation of the principles of mixed model analysis has been limited to relatively simple models in which only one independent variable was analysed. In this chapter the models to be analysed will be extended with some covariates. In the example a study will be used in which the researchers were interested in the relationship between overweight and quality of life among individuals aged between 30 and 60 years. The study was performed with subjects from different cities, and there was an over-sampling of individuals with overweight. Table 7.1 shows the descriptive information regarding the example dataset.

The first analysis to be performed is a mixed model analysis with quality of life as the outcome, overweight as the independent variable and a random intercept on city level. Output 7.1 shows the result of this analysis.

From the first part of Output 7.1 it can be seen that there are 29 cities in the example dataset and that the number of subjects within a city range between 5 and 24.

Regarding the analysis, from the last line in Output 7.1 it can be seen that a random intercept is necessary. The likelihood ratio test comparing the model with a random intercept on city level and the naive linear regression model in which the clustering on city level is ignored gives a p-value of 0.0014, which is highly significant. The regression coefficient for overweight (-5.136096) indicates that for the subjects with overweight quality of life is 5.1 points lower than for the subjects with normal weight. The confidence interval ranges between -8.2 to -2.0 and the corresponding p-value = 0.001.

Table 7.1 Descriptive information regarding the example dataset

	Mean	Standard deviation
Quality of life	59.8	12.8
Age	50.1	5.7
	Percentage	
Overweight (yes/no)	77.1%/22.9%	
Gender (females/males)	50.3%/49.7%	
City size (small/big)	46.7%/53.3%	

Output 7.1 Result of a linear mixed model analysis of the relationship between overweight and quality of life with a random intercept on city level

```
Mixed-effects ML regression              Number of obs    =      366
Group variable: city                     Number of groups =       29

                                         Obs per group:
                                                        min =        5
                                                        avg =     12.6
                                                        max =       24

                                         Wald chi2(1)     =    10.52
Log likelihood =  -1442.312              Prob > chi2      =   0.0012

------------------------------------------------------------------------
     qol |    Coef.    Std. Err.      z    P>|z|    [95% Conf. Interval]
---------+--------------------------------------------------------------
overweight | -5.136096  1.583497   -3.24  0.001   -8.239692   -2.0325
    _cons | 64.08707   1.549981   41.35  0.000    61.04917   67.12498
------------------------------------------------------------------------

------------------------------------------------------------------------
 Random-effects Parameters  |  Estimate  Std. Err.    [95% Conf. Interval]
----------------------------+-------------------------------------------
city: Identity              |
              var(_cons)    | 13.57602   7.336871    4.70716    39.15491
----------------------------+-------------------------------------------
            var(Residual)   | 146.0693   11.30141    125.5166   169.9873
------------------------------------------------------------------------
LR test vs. linear model: chibar2(01) = 8.93    Prob >= chibar2 = 0.0014
```

Theoretically, the next step is to add a random slope for overweight on city level to the model. However, adding a random slope for overweight to the model led to problems in the estimation of the standard errors of the random part of the model, and besides that, it did not improve the model. So, the model with only a random intercept on city level will be used as starting point for the next step in the modelling procedure.

The regression coefficient reported in Output 7.1 is mostly referred to as the crude result of the analysis. In the example dataset there are several

Output 7.2 Result of a linear mixed model analysis of the relationship between overweight and quality of life adjusted for gender with a random intercept on city level

```
Mixed-effects ML regression                    Number of obs    =        366
Group variable: city                           Number of groups =         29

                                               Obs per group:
                                                          min =          5
                                                          avg =       12.6
                                                          max =         24

                                               Wald chi2(2)     =      10.83
Log likelihood = -1442.1628                    Prob > chi2      =     0.0044

------------------------------------------------------------------------------
        qol |     Coef.   Std. Err.      z    P>|z|     [95% Conf. Interval]
------------+-----------------------------------------------------------------
 overweight | -5.171901    1.58415    -3.26   0.001    -8.276778   -2.067024
     gender | -.7025328   1.285565    -0.55   0.585    -3.222194    1.817128
      _cons |  64.46349    1.69494    38.03   0.000     61.14147    67.78551
------------------------------------------------------------------------------

------------------------------------------------------------------------------
  Random-effects Parameters  |   Estimate   Std. Err.    [95% Conf. Interval]
-----------------------------+------------------------------------------------
city: Identity               |
                 var(_cons)  |   13.63958   7.360371     4.736576    39.27694
-----------------------------+------------------------------------------------
               var(Residual) |   145.916    11.29078     125.3829    169.8118
------------------------------------------------------------------------------
LR test vs. linear model: chibar2(01) = 8.97        Prob >= chibar2 = 0.0014
```

variables available that perhaps influence this relationship. In the next step of the modelling procedure it is investigated whether the relationship between overweight and quality of life is influenced by (1) gender and (2) age. Output 7.2 shows the result of the analysis adjusted for gender.

From Output 7.2 it can be seen that the relationship between quality of life and overweight is not influence by gender. The regression coefficient for overweight changes from −5.14 in the crude analysis to −5.17 in the adjusted analysis. Theoretically it would be possible to add a random slope for gender on city level to the model, but to avoid unnecessary complexity, mostly random slopes for covariates are not added to the model. Nevertheless, Output 7.3 shows the result of an analysis in which a random slope for gender on city level is added to the model.

When a likelihood ratio test is performed to compare the models with and without a random slope for gender (and of course the covariance between the random intercept and the random slope), it can be seen that there is no significant improvement of the model: the difference between the $-2 \log$ likelihood of the model without a random slope ($-2 \times -1442.1628 = 2884.3$) and the model with a random slope for gender ($-2 \times -1440.136 = 2880.3$)

Output 7.3 Result of a linear mixed model analysis of the relationship between overweight and quality of life adjusted for gender with a random intercept and a random slope for gender on city level

```
Mixed-effects ML regression                Number of obs      =       366
Group variable: city                       Number of groups   =        29

                                           Obs per group:
                                                         min =         5
                                                         avg =      12.6
                                                         max =        24

                                           Wald chi2(2)       =     11.06
Log likelihood = -1440.136                 Prob > chi2        =    0.0040

-----------------------------------------------------------------------------
        qol |     Coef.   Std. Err.      z    P>|z|     [95% Conf. Interval]
------------+----------------------------------------------------------------
 overweight | -5.145635   1.560384    -3.30   0.001    -8.203932   -2.087338
     gender | -.7951039   1.597302    -0.50   0.619    -3.925759    2.335551
      _cons |   64.4717   1.792239    35.97   0.000     60.95897    67.98442
-----------------------------------------------------------------------------

-----------------------------------------------------------------------------
  Random-effects Parameters  |   Estimate   Std. Err.     [95% Conf. Interval]
-----------------------------+-----------------------------------------------
city: Unstructured           |
              var(gender)    |   25.28435   18.82056      5.878338    108.7549
              var(_cons)     |   25.20169   12.64653      9.425099     67.3866
          cov(gender,_cons)  |  -18.6632    13.04194     -44.22493    6.898522
-----------------------------+-----------------------------------------------
            var(Residual)    |   139.7986   11.19523      119.4917    163.5566
-----------------------------------------------------------------------------
LR test vs. linear model: chi2(3) = 13.02              Prob > chi2 = 0.0046
```

equals 4, and on a Chi-square distribution with 2 degrees of freedom, this difference is not statistically significant (i.e. lower than the critical value of 5.99). Note again, that in real-life practice random slopes for potential covariates are seldom investigated; only a random slope for the independent variable of interest is added to the model if necessary.

So, it can be concluded that gender is not influencing the relationship between overweight and quality of life in this study. The next potential influencing variable to be considered is age. Output 7.4 shows the result of the analysis adjusted for age.

When age is added to the model, the regression coefficient for overweight changes from −5.1 to −2.7; obviously, part of the relationship between overweight and quality of life is caused by age. From the sign of the regression coefficient for age it can be seen that higher age is associated with higher quality of life. So, the average age of subjects with overweight must be lower than the average age of subjects without overweight. When looking at the average ages for the two groups it can be seen that indeed is true; the average age for the subjects without overweight is 52.1, while the

Output 7.4 Result of a linear mixed model analysis of the relationship between overweight and quality of life adjusted for age with a random intercept on city level

```
Mixed-effects ML regression                    Number of obs    =        366
Group variable: city                           Number of groups =         29

                                               Obs per group:
                                                            min =          5
                                                            avg =       12.6
                                                            max =         24

                                               Wald chi2(2)     =     121.27
Log likelihood = -1395.2384                    Prob > chi2      =     0.0000
------------------------------------------------------------------------------
         qol |      Coef.   Std. Err.      z    P>|z|     [95% Conf. Interval]
-------------+----------------------------------------------------------------
  overweight |  -2.713377   1.412475    -1.92   0.055    -5.481778     .0550235
         age |    1.07688    .1038617   10.37   0.000     .8733145    1.280445
       _cons |   8.252211   5.566652     1.48   0.138    -2.658226    19.16265
------------------------------------------------------------------------------

------------------------------------------------------------------------------
  Random-effects Parameters  |   Estimate   Std. Err.    [95% Conf. Interval]
-----------------------------+------------------------------------------------
city: Identity               |
                 var(_cons)  |   12.44881   5.988728     4.848885    31.96052
-----------------------------+------------------------------------------------
               var(Residual) |   112.0853   8.645208     96.35963    130.3774
------------------------------------------------------------------------------
LR test vs. linear model: chibar2(01) = 12.39         Prob >= chibar2 = 0.0002
```

average age for the subjects with overweight is 49.5. From Output 7.4 it can also be seen that age is highly significant related to quality of life. The fact that a particular covariate is significantly related to the outcome variable does not indicate directly that the particular covariate also influences the relationship between the two variables. Therefore, the covariate must also be related to the independent variable. Suppose that the average age in the normal weight group and the overweight group were exactly the same, age could never influence the relationship between overweight and quality of life. This has to do with the definition of confounding. A covariate can only be a confounder in a particular relationship when the covariate is related to the outcome and related to the independent variable. It is important that in this definition it is not said that those relationships must be significant. Whether a relationship is significant or not, is not really a big deal in this respect.

Both age and gender are variables measured on the level of the subject. When there is clustering in the data, it is also possible that variables that are measured on a higher level are influencing the relationship of interest. In the example dataset, the variable size of the city is, of course, measured on

Output 7.5 Result of a linear mixed model analysis of the relationship between overweight and quality of life adjusted for city size with a random intercept on city level

```
Mixed-effects ML regression                    Number of obs     =       366
Group variable: city                           Number of groups  =        29

                                               Obs per group:
                                                           min =         5
                                                           avg =      12.6
                                                           max =        24

                                               Wald chi2(2)      =     10.64
Log likelihood = -1442.252                     Prob > chi2       =    0.0049

------------------------------------------------------------------------------
      qol |      Coef.   Std. Err.      z     P>|z|     [95% Conf. Interval]
----------+-------------------------------------------------------------------
overweight | -5.125015   1.583552    -3.24    0.001    -8.228719    -2.021311
 city_size | -.6650066   1.919313    -0.35    0.729    -4.426792     3.096778
     _cons |  64.45283    1.87539    34.37    0.000     60.77714     68.12853
------------------------------------------------------------------------------


------------------------------------------------------------------------------
 Random-effects Parameters  |   Estimate   Std. Err.     [95% Conf. Interval]
----------------------------+-------------------------------------------------
city: Identity              |
                var(_cons)  |   13.56279    7.30328      4.720577     38.96757
----------------------------+-------------------------------------------------
              var(Residual) |   146.0254   11.29408      125.4855     169.9273
------------------------------------------------------------------------------
LR test vs. linear model: chibar2(01) = 9.01          Prob >= chibar2 = 0.0013
```

city level. It is interesting to investigate whether the relationship between overweight and quality of life is influenced by the size of the city. Output 7.5 shows the result of this analysis.

From Output 7.5 it can be seen that the size of the city is not influencing the relationship between overweight and quality of life. The regression coefficient for overweight is not different from the crude regression coefficient reported in Output 7.1.

It should be realized that the procedure to investigate the influence of covariates on a particular relationship described in this section is not really different than the procedure used in standard (linear) regression analysis.

The same goes for the investigation of possible effect modification. The way this is done in mixed model analysis is exactly the same as it is done in standard (linear) regression analysis: by adding an interaction term (i.e. a multiplication of the variable of interest and the potential effect modifier) and the potential effect modifier to the model. Suppose there is interest in the question whether the relationship between overweight and quality of life is different for males and females. To investigate this possible effect

Output 7.6 Result of a linear mixed model analysis of the relationship between overweight and quality of life, with an interaction with gender and with a random intercept on city level

```
Mixed-effects ML regression                    Number of obs    =       366
Group variable: city                           Number of groups =        29

                                               Obs per group:
                                                           min =         5
                                                           avg =      12.6
                                                           max =        24

                                               Wald chi2(3)     =     13.90
Log likelihood = -1440.6903                    Prob > chi2      =    0.0030
```

qol	Coef.	Std. Err.	z	P>|z|	[95% Conf. Interval]	
overweight						
overweight	-7.862615	2.21964	-3.54	0.000	-12.21303	-3.5122
gender						
males	-4.728757	2.667006	-1.77	0.076	-9.955993	.4984792
overweight#						
gender						
overweight #						
males	5.214576	3.031157	1.72	0.085	-.7263821	11.15553
_cons	66.5577	2.080994	31.98	0.000	62.47903	70.63638

Random-effects Parameters	Estimate	Std. Err.	[95% Conf. Interval]	
city: Identity				
var(_cons)	13.91076	7.363824	4.92898	39.25947
var(Residual)	144.5738	11.18127	124.2391	168.2369

```
LR test vs. linear model: chibar2(01) = 9.48          Prob >= chibar2 = 0.0010
```

modification, the interaction between gender and overweight is added to the model. Output 7.6 shows the result of this analysis.

In the fixed part of the regression model shown in Output 7.6, three regression coefficients are given: one for overweight, one for gender and one for the interaction between overweight and gender. Although the interpretation of the regression coefficients is exactly the same as the interpretation of the regression coefficients of a standard regression analysis with an interaction term, it is worthwhile to discuss the interpretation of the three regression coefficients. The regression coefficient for overweight (-7.86) is still the difference in quality of life between subjects with overweight and subjects without overweight. However, when an interaction term is in the model, this difference does not hold for the whole population, but only for the subjects who have the value zero for the effect modifier. The effect modifier in this particular situation is gender and gender is coded zero for females, so the regression coefficient for overweight is the difference in quality of life between overweight females and normal weight females. What is then the difference in quality of life between overweight males and normal weight males? That difference can be obtained by summing the regression coefficient for overweight and the regression coefficient for the interaction term, $-7.86 + 5.21 = -2.65$. The same regression coefficient can be obtained from an analysis in which gender is recoded (0 for males and 1 for females). Output 7.7 shows the result of the analysis with the recoded gender variable.

Based on the two analyses it is obvious that the regression coefficient of the interaction term reflects the difference in relationship between overweight and quality of life between males and females. That difference in

Output 7.7 Result of a linear mixed model analysis of the relationship between overweight and quality of life, with an interaction with gender (recoded) and with a random intercept on city level

```
Mixed-effects ML regression              Number of obs    =        366
Group variable: city                     Number of groups =         29

                                         Obs per group:
                                                       min =          5
                                                       avg =       12.6
                                                       max =         24

                                         Wald chi2(3)     =      13.90
Log likelihood = -1440.6903              Prob > chi2      =     0.0030
```

qol	Coef.	Std. Err.	z	P>|z|	[95% Conf. Interval]	
overweight						
overweight	-2.64804	2.156527	-1.23	0.219	-6.874755	1.578676
gender						
females	4.728757	2.667006	1.77	0.076	-.4984792	9.955993
overweight#						
gender						
overweight #						
females	-5.214576	3.031157	-1.72	0.085	-11.15553	.7263821
_cons	61.82894	2.00689	30.81	0.000	57.89551	65.76238

Random-effects Parameters	Estimate	Std. Err.	[95% Conf. Interval]	
city: Identity				
var(_cons)	13.91076	7.363824	4.92898	39.25947
var(Residual)	144.5738	11.18127	124.2391	168.2369

```
LR test vs. linear model: chibar2(01) = 9.48          Prob >= chibar2 = 0.0010
```

relationship is −5.21, but from Output 7.6 and Output 7.7 it can be seen that this difference in relationship is not statistically significant. It should be noted, though, that sometimes for interaction terms a *p*-value of 0.10 is considered as a cut-off for significance (see Section 7.2.2).

A special feature of mixed model analysis is that so-called cross-level interactions can be analysed. A cross-level interaction indicates an interaction between a variable measured on a lower level and a variable measured on a higher level. The way this is done in mixed model analysis is exactly the same as for interaction terms in standard analysis. In the example, for instance, the cross-level interaction between overweight and the size of the city can be investigated. Output 7.8 shows the result of the analysis that includes this cross-level interaction.

Output 7.8 Result of a linear mixed model analysis of the relationship between overweight and quality of life, with a cross-level interaction with city size and with a random intercept on city level

```
Mixed-effects ML regression                    Number of obs    =         366
Group variable: city                           Number of groups =          29

                                               Obs per group:
                                                           min =           5
                                                           avg =        12.6
                                                           max =          24

                                               Wald chi2(3)     =       11.71
Log likelihood = -1441.7378                    Prob > chi2      =      0.0084

------------------------------------------------------------------------------
         qol |     Coef.   Std. Err.      z    P>|z|    [95% Conf. Interval]
-------------+----------------------------------------------------------------
  overweight |
  overweight |  -3.413385   2.313185   -1.48   0.140    -7.947144    1.120375
             |
   city_size |
         big |   1.810705   3.106799    0.58   0.560    -4.278509    7.899919
             |
 overweight#|
   city_size |
 overweight #|
         big |  -3.217149   3.169474   -1.02   0.310    -9.429204    2.994906
             |
       _cons |   63.15748   2.271821   27.80   0.000     58.70479   67.61017
------------------------------------------------------------------------------

------------------------------------------------------------------------------
  Random-effects Parameters |   Estimate   Std. Err.    [95% Conf. Interval]
----------------------------+-------------------------------------------------
city: Identity              |
             var(_cons)     |   13.67446     7.2788      4.81751   38.81482
----------------------------+-------------------------------------------------
            var(Residual)   |   145.5471    11.25102     125.0848   169.3569
------------------------------------------------------------------------------
LR test vs. linear model: chibar2(01) = 9.30          Prob >= chibar2 = 0.0011
```

From Output 7.8 it can be seen that the relationship between overweight and quality of life is stronger in big cities (-3.4 for small cities and -6.6 [$-3.4 + -3.2$] for big cities), but that this difference is not statistically significant (the p-value of the interaction term equals 0.31).

7.2 Prediction Models and Association Models

7.2.1 Introduction

When performing a multivariable analysis, it is extremely important to realise what kind of question should be answered with the multivariable analysis. This not only applies to multivariable mixed model analysis, but basically to all multivariable analyses. Within multivariable analysis a distinction should be made between prediction or prognostic models and association models. With association models (Section 7.2.2) the research question of interest concerns the association between one main or central independent variable (or a small set of central independent variables) and a certain outcome. The general idea behind association models is to estimate this relationship or association as accurately as possible. This means that adjusting for confounding and/or possible effect modification must be taken into account. For prediction or prognostic models (Section 7.2.3) the research question (and therefore the modelling strategy) is different. Constructing a prediction model involves searching for the best, most simple, combination of independent variables to predict a certain outcome. It should be realised that each of the modelling strategies applied in the following sections of this chapter are examples of possible strategies.

7.2.2 Association Models

The modelling procedure described in Section 7.1 is basically the construction of an association model. The main or central determinant in the analysis was overweight, and the relationship between overweight and quality of life was adjusted for gender, age and city size. This was done in separate analyses for the potential confounders. In fact, the way association models are constructed within mixed model analysis is more or less the same as the way in which association models are constructed in standard regression analysis. Probably the most common example of constructing an association model is when the effect of a certain intervention is evaluated. The main or central determinant is the intervention, and the effect of this central determinant has to be estimated as accurately as possible. This means that, when necessary, the effect of the intervention has to be adjusted for potential confounders, and that possible effect modification has to be taken into account.

Therefore, in this section a randomised controlled trial (RCT) will be used as an example for the construction of an association model. The intervention is applied with the intention of lowering cholesterol concentration in the blood. The intervention is applied at the patient level, and the patients are randomly allocated into the intervention group and a control group; 131 patients were allocated to the intervention group and 145 to the control group. Furthermore, patients from 10 general practitioners (GPs) were involved in this study. The patients were measured at baseline (before the start of the intervention) and directly after the intervention ended. In addition to the outcome variable cholesterol, measured directly after the intervention period, there is also information available with regard to the baseline value of cholesterol, age, BMI, smoking behaviour and gender. Table 7.2 shows the descriptive information regarding the dataset used in this example.

The first step in the construction of an association model is to perform a crude analysis. In a crude analysis, only the main central determinant (i.e. the intervention variable) is present in the model. However, in the analysis of the effect of a certain intervention (evaluated in an RCT) it is important to adjust for possible differences in the outcome variable at baseline (Twisk and Proper, 2004; Twisk, 2013). This analysis, which is known as analysis of

Table 7.2 Descriptive information regarding the example dataset

	Mean	Standard deviation
Cholesterol (mmol/l)	5.96	0.93
Baseline cholesterol (mmol/l)	6.34	0.93
BMI	31.2	5.8
Age (years)	39.3	7.1
	Percentage	
Smoking (yes/no)	35.5%/64.5%	
Gender (females/males)	56.9%/43.1%	

covariance, is necessary to adjust for the phenomenon of regression to the mean, which can occur when the intervention group and the control group differ from each other with respect to the outcome variable measured at baseline. Furthermore, the patients are clustered within GPs, so, in the first analysis, a random intercept on GP level is added to the model. Output 7.9 shows the result of the crude analysis.

From the last line in Output 7.9 it can be seen that a random intercept on GP level is necessary. The likelihood ratio test to compare the model without a random intercept to the model with a random intercept provides a highly significant p-value (the difference between the two $-2 \log$ likelihoods equals 15.53). The next step in the modelling procedure is to add a random slope for the intervention on a GP level to the model. Because the randomisation is performed on patient level, a random slope for the intervention variable is possible. It should be realised that in a study in which the randomisation is performed on GP level, a random slope for the intervention variable would not have been possible (see Section 2.8.1). Output 7.10 shows the result of the analysis, including a random slope for the intervention variable.

Output 7.9 Result of a linear mixed model analysis performed to determine the effect of an intervention on cholesterol adjusted for the baseline cholesterol value with a random intercept on GP level

```
Mixed-effects ML regression                  Number of obs    =      276
Group variable: GP                           Number of groups =       10

                                             Obs per group:
                                                        min =         21
                                                        avg =       27.6
                                                        max =         35

                                             Wald chi2(2)     =     84.37
Log likelihood = -283.73987                  Prob > chi2      =    0.0000
```

cholesterol	Coef.	Std. Err.	z	P>|z|	[95% Conf. Interval]	
intervention	-.0445694	.0843894	-0.53	0.597	-.2099696	.1208308
base_chol	.473225	.0524235	9.03	0.000	.3704768	.5759733
_cons	3.006144	.3435256	8.75	0.000	2.332846	3.679442

Random-effects Parameters	Estimate	Std. Err.	[95% Conf. Interval]	
GP: Identity				
var(_cons)	.0943905	.0555077	.0298103	.2988753
var(Residual)	.4262952	.03715	.3593614	.505696

```
LR test vs. linear model: chibar2(01) = 15.53        Prob >= chibar2 = 0.0000
```

Output 7.10 Result of a linear mixed model analysis performed to determine the effect of an intervention on cholesterol adjusted for the baseline cholesterol value with a random intercept and a random slope for the intervention on GP level

```
Mixed-effects ML regression                    Number of obs     =        276
Group variable: GP                             Number of groups  =         10

                                               Obs per group:
                                                            min =         21
                                                            avg =       27.6
                                                            max =         35

                                               Wald chi2(2)      =      33.19
Log likelihood = -264.11924                    Prob > chi2       =     0.0000

-----------------------------------------------------------------------------
 cholesterol |     Coef.   Std. Err.      z    P>|z|    [95% Conf. Interval]
-------------+---------------------------------------------------------------
intervention |  -.0742738   .2108757    -0.35   0.725   -.4875826     .339035
   base_chol |   .3057169   .0530722     5.76   0.000    .2016972    .4097365
       _cons |   4.048716   .3854034    10.51   0.000     3.29334    4.804093
-----------------------------------------------------------------------------


-----------------------------------------------------------------------------
  Random-effects Parameters  |   Estimate   Std. Err.    [95% Conf. Interval]
-----------------------------+-----------------------------------------------
GP: Unstructured             |
              var(interv~n)  |   .3874251   .2036165      .1383016    1.085296
               var(_cons)    |    .380226   .1890792      .1434681    1.007693
          cov(interv~n,_cons)|  -.3705016   .1892897     -.7415027    .0004995
-----------------------------+-----------------------------------------------
              var(Residual)  |   .3502633   .0312319      .2941004    .4171513
-----------------------------------------------------------------------------
LR test vs. linear model: chi2(3) = 54.78               Prob > chi2 = 0.0000
```

Based on the likelihood ratio test it can be concluded that a random slope for the intervention variable is necessary. The difference between the −2 log likelihoods is 39.3: $-2 \times -283.73987 = 567.5$ for the model with only a random intercept and $-2 \times -264.11924 = 528.2$ for the model with a random intercept, a random slope for the intervention variable and the covariance between the random intercept and random slope. This is (evaluated on a Chi-square distribution with 2 degrees of freedom) highly significant. So, the crude intervention effect can be derived from the analysis with both a random intercept and a random slope for the intervention variable on GP level (Output 7.10). This intervention effect (−0.074) indicates that, adjusted for the differences at baseline, the cholesterol concentration in the intervention group is 0.074 mmol/l lower than the cholesterol concentration in the control group. This small difference has a 95% confidence interval that ranges between −0.48 and 0.34 and has a corresponding p-value of 0.73.

The next step in the modelling procedure is to adjust for (all) potential confounders. However, it should be realised that in a situation in which there are many potential confounders in comparison to the number of subjects in the study, an analysis with all potential confounders is impossible. When this is the case, only important confounders can be added to the model. The importance of a potential confounder is often evaluated by the change in the magnitude of the regression coefficient of the main determinant. The greater the change, the more important that potential confounder is. It is sometimes argued that only potential confounders that lead to a change of 10% or more in the magnitude of the regression coefficient should be added to the final adjusted model. However, like all other cut-off values in statistics, this cut-off value is highly arbitrary. The difference between mixed model analysis and standard regression analysis in this second step of the modelling procedure is the fact that in mixed model analysis the necessity of a random slope can also be evaluated for the potential confounders. However, as has been mentioned before, in real-life practice, random slopes for the potential confounders are mostly not taken into account. Output 7.11 shows the result of the analysis adjusting for all potential confounders present in the example dataset (i.e. age, BMI, smoking and gender).

From Output 7.11 it can be seen that the adjustment for all potential confounders has some influence on the magnitude of the intervention effect (i.e. the regression coefficient for the intervention variable). The intervention effect changes from -0.074 to -0.119 and, although the magnitude of the standard error decreases from 0.21 to 0.12, the intervention effect is still not significant (p-value = 0.302).

When reporting the results of an intervention study or an association model in general, it is strongly recommended that the results of both the crude and the adjusted analysis are reported. Table 7.3 shows the results of the analyses performed on the example dataset.

From Table 7.3 it can be seen that no information is provided about the random intercept variance and the random slope variance of the intervention variable. This is not strange, because the only interest is in the effect of the intervention. The reason for using mixed model analysis is that the correlated observations within the GP must be taken into account in the most efficient way. It should be noted that the recommendation to report

Output 7.11 Result of a linear mixed model analysis performed to determine the effect of an intervention on cholesterol adjusted for the baseline cholesterol value and other covariates with a random intercept and a random slope for the intervention on GP level

```
Mixed-effects ML regression                    Number of obs    =      276
Group variable: GP                             Number of groups =       10

                                               Obs per group:
                                                          min =       21
                                                          avg =     27.6
                                                          max =       35

                                               Wald chi2(6)     =   129.66
Log likelihood = -233.60771                    Prob > chi2      =   0.0000

------------------------------------------------------------------------------
cholesterol |    Coef.   Std. Err.     z    P>|z|    [95% Conf. Interval]
------------+-----------------------------------------------------------------
intervention| -.1192816  .1155315   -1.03   0.302   -.3457192    .107156
 base_chol  |  .2150226  .0504958    4.26   0.000    .1160527   .3139925
       age  |  .0440574  .0077901    5.66   0.000     .028789   .0593258
       bmi  |  .0427494   .011483    3.72   0.000    .0202431   .0652557
    smoking | -.2763769  .1129454   -2.45   0.014   -.4977459  -.0550079
     gender | -.0662697  .1141981   -0.58   0.562   -.2900938   .1575544
      _cons |  1.729768  .4520865    3.83   0.000    .8436944   2.615841
------------------------------------------------------------------------------

------------------------------------------------------------------------------
Random-effects Parameters    | Estimate   Std. Err.    [95% Conf. Interval]
-----------------------------+------------------------------------------------
GP: Unstructured             |
               var(interv~n) |  .0818521  .0633502     .017957       .3731
                 var(_cons)  |  .2422039  .1225155    .0898695    .6527542
          cov(interv~n,_cons)| -.1199308  .081613    -.2798894    .0400278
-----------------------------+------------------------------------------------
               var(Residual) |  .2816549  .0249769    .2367193    .3351205
------------------------------------------------------------------------------
LR test vs. linear model: chi2(3) = 49.82               Prob > chi2 = 0.0000
```

Table 7.3 Results of a linear mixed model analysis to determine the effect of an intervention on cholesterol

	Regression coefficient[1]	95% confidence interval	p-value
Crude	−0.074	−0.488 to 0.339	0.73
Adjusted[2]	−0.119	−0.346 to 0.107	0.30

[1] Regression coefficient indicates the difference in cholesterol between the intervention and the control group at the end of the intervention period, adjusted for baseline cholesterol values.

[2] Adjusted for BMI, smoking, gender and age.

both the crude and the adjusted results does not only apply to mixed model analysis, but also for all other statistical analysis.

Another important aspect in the building of association models is the evaluation of potential effect modification. It can, for instance, be important to determine whether the intervention effect is different for males and females. Potential effect modification can be investigated by adding interaction terms to the model. As has been mentioned before, an interaction term consists of a multiplication of the main determinant and the potential effect modifier, and when the regression coefficient of the interaction term is statistically significant, it indicates that the effect of the intervention is significantly different for the different values of the effect modifier. Because the analysis with an interaction term has less power, the significance levels of interaction terms are usually set slightly higher than 0.05 (e.g. p-values < 0.10).

To investigate potential effect modification in the example dataset, the crude analysis that was presented in Output 7.10 will be used. In general, the way to investigate potential effect modification is to add each interaction term separately to the model. When this procedure is followed for the four covariates in the example dataset, it can be seen that only the interaction with smoking behaviour is statistically significant (p-value = 0.012). Output 7.12 shows the result of this analysis.

So, the result of the analysis with interaction terms shows that the effect of the intervention is significantly different for smokers and non-smokers. The implication of this significant interaction is that the effects of the intervention should also be reported separately for smokers and non-smokers. It has been mentioned before in the discussion about confounding that it is recommended to report the results of both a crude analysis and an adjusted analysis. So, in this situation, with a significant interaction between the intervention and smoking, a crude result and an adjusted result should (also) be reported for smokers and for non-smokers. Both can be obtained by performing stratified analyses for smokers and non-smokers, but it is more elegant to use the analysis with the interaction term. Because non-smokers are coded as zero, the intervention effect, the 95% CI and the p-value for non-smokers can be obtained from Output 7.12. The intervention effect (and 95% CI and p-value) for smokers can be obtained by reanalysing the data with a recoded smoking variable (coding the

Output 7.12 Result of a linear mixed model analysis performed to determine the effect of an intervention on cholesterol adjusted for the baseline cholesterol value, with an interaction with smoking and with a random intercept and a random slope for the intervention on GP level

```
Mixed-effects ML regression                    Number of obs    =        276
Group variable: GP                             Number of groups =         10

                                               Obs per group:
                                                            min =         21
                                                            avg =       27.6
                                                            max =         35

                                               Wald chi2(4)     =      45.16
Log likelihood = -259.27747                    Prob > chi2      =     0.0000
```

cholesterol	Coef.	Std. Err.	z	P>|z|	[95% Conf. Interval]	
intervention						
intervent~n	.0955751	.1967426	0.49	0.627	-.2900332	.4811835
smoking						
smoking	.3537535	.1131344	3.13	0.002	.1320142	.5754928
intervention#|						
smoking						
intervent~n #|						
smoking	-.4247202	.1686332	-2.52	0.012	-.7552352	-.0942052
base_chol	.3013933	.0524874	5.74	0.000	.1985199	.4042668
_cons	3.934343	.3723429	10.57	0.000	3.204565	4.664122

Random-effects Parameters	Estimate	Std. Err.	[95% Conf. Interval]	
GP: Unstructured				
var(interv~n)	.2954493	.1649831	.0988917	.8826857
var(_cons)	.3033835	.1556858	.1109648	.8294662
cov(interv~n,_cons)	-.2831674	.1530287	-.5830981	.0167632
var(Residual)	.3391667	.0302963	.2846944	.4040615

```
LR test vs. linear model: chi2(3) = 41.19                  Prob > chi2 = 0.0000
```

smokers as zero). Output 7.13 shows the result of the analysis with the recoded smoking variable.

Table 7.4 summarises the results of the analyses with smoking as an effect modifier.

From the results that are summarised in Table 7.4, it can be seen that there is a highly significant intervention effect for smokers, and that this effect is only significant when an adjustment has been made for age, BMI and gender. Apparently, for non-smokers the intervention does not have an effect. In fact, the positive regression coefficient observed for non-smokers indicates that, adjusted for the baseline value of cholesterol, the intervention group has higher cholesterol values after the intervention, compared to the control group.

Output 7.13 Result of a linear mixed model analysis performed to determine the effect of an intervention on cholesterol adjusted for the baseline cholesterol value, with an interaction with smoking (recoded) and with a random intercept and a random slope for the intervention on GP level

```
Mixed-effects ML regression              Number of obs     =        276
Group variable: GP                       Number of groups  =         10

                                         Obs per group:
                                                       min =         21
                                                       avg =       27.6
                                                       max =         35

                                         Wald chi2(4)      =      45.16
Log likelihood = -259.27747              Prob > chi2       =     0.0000

-------------------------------------------------------------------------------
  cholesterol |    Coef.    Std. Err.     z     P>|z|    [95% Conf. Interval]
--------------+----------------------------------------------------------------
 intervention |
  intervent~n | -.3291451   .2172327   -1.52   0.130   -.7549134    .0966233
              |
      smoking |
  non smoking | -.3537535   .1131344   -3.13   0.002   -.5754928   -.1320142
              |
 intervention#|
      smoking |
 intervent~n #|
  non smoking |  .4247202   .1686332    2.52   0.012    .0942052    .7552352
              |
    base_chol |  .3013933   .0524874    5.74   0.000    .1985199    .4042668
        _cons |  4.288097   .3818048   11.23   0.000   3.539773    5.036421
-------------------------------------------------------------------------------

-------------------------------------------------------------------------------
  Random-effects Parameters  |   Estimate   Std. Err.    [95% Conf. Interval]
-----------------------------+-------------------------------------------------
GP: Unstructured             |
            var(interv~n)    |  .2954493   .1649831     .0988917    .8826857
              var(_cons)     |  .3033835   .1556858     .1109648    .8294662
        cov(interv~n,_cons)  | -.2831674   .1530287    -.5830981    .0167632
-----------------------------+-------------------------------------------------
            var(Residual)    |  .3391667   .0302963     .2846944    .4040615
-------------------------------------------------------------------------------
LR test vs. linear model: chi2(3) = 41.19                  Prob > chi2 = 0.0000
```

It should be noted that in the present analysis a significant interaction was found for a dichotomous variable (i.e. smoking). For the different groups of the dichotomous variable (i.e. smokers and non-smokers), separate results can be reported. When a significant interaction is found with a continuous variable (e.g. age or BMI), the situation is slightly more complicated. There are basically two possibilities that are often used in this situation. The first possibility is to create two or more groups for the continuous variable and to estimate separate intervention effects for the different groups. However, the disadvantage of this method is that grouping a continuous variable not only leads to a loss of information, but it leads to

Table 7.4 Regression coefficients, 95% confidence intervals and *p*-values for the effect of a cholesterol-lowering intervention for smokers and non-smokers. Both crude and adjusted[1] results are presented

	Regression coefficient	95% confidence interval	*p*-value
Non-smokers			
Crude	0.10	−0.29 to 0.48	0.63
Adjusted[1]	0.07	−0.13 to 0.28	0.47
Smokers			
Crude	−0.33	−0.75 to 0.10	0.13
Adjusted[1]	−0.43	−0.68 to −0.19	<0.01

[1] Adjusted for age, BMI and gender.

a different variable. Another possibility is to report the average intervention effect that can be obtained from an analysis without the interaction term, and report that a significant interaction was found with a particular continuous variable. Furthermore, it should be mentioned that this interaction has to be interpreted in such a way that the intervention effect is stronger or weaker when the value of the continuous effect modifier is higher. Whether the effect is stronger or weaker depends on the sign of the regression coefficient for the intervention variable and the sign of the regression coefficient of the interaction term.

7.2.3 Prediction or Prognostic Models

The general idea underlying the building of a prediction or prognostic model is that, given a certain set of independent variables, the best and most simple model (i.e. combination of independent variables) is built to predict the outcome variable of interest. In general, there are two strategies that can be followed: a forward selection procedure or a backward selection procedure.

A forward selection starts by adding the independent variable that is most strongly associated with the outcome variable to the model. This starting model is then extended with the second best predictor, then with the third best predictor, and so on, until a predefined end-point is reached. This end-point can be that all variables included in the model must have a significant association with the outcome, but sometimes the cut-off value is somewhat higher (e.g. all variables with p-values < 0.10 are allowed in the model).With a backward selection procedure, the starting point is a model with all possible predictor variables. The modelling procedure starts by removing the independent variable that is least strongly associated with the outcome variable and carries on removing these variables until it ends when a certain predefined end-point is reached.

Although for standard regression analysis mostly automatic forward and backward selection procedures are available, for mixed model analysis these automatic forward and backward selection procedures are not available, so all modelling must be done manually. Within a mixed model setting, however, not only is the significance of the independent variables important, but also the random part of that relationship can be of importance. There are a few ways in which to construct a prediction or prognostic model, and unfortunately different modelling strategies do not always produce the same results. In the literature it is sometimes argued that in mixed model analysis a backward strategy is preferred, and that one should start the modelling procedure with a full model. A full model is then defined as a model with not only all independent variables, but also all possible random variance components. Theoretically this is probably the best approach that can be followed, but in practice it is not possible unless there is a very large study population and only a few potential predictors. In most situations, however, the coefficients of such a full model cannot be estimated. Therefore, an alternative approach must be followed.

In the next part of this chapter, an example will be given of an alternative strategy that can be followed to construct a prediction (or prognostic) model. It should be realised that this is just one of the possibilities; there are, of course, many more strategies available.

In the example dataset, systolic blood pressure is the outcome variable of interest, and the potential predictor variables are age, gender, BMI, smoking, alcohol consumption and physical activity. Smoking is a dichotomous variable, while alcohol consumption and physical activity are categorised into three groups. For alcohol consumption the first group consists of the non-drinkers, the second group are the moderate drinkers and the third group are the heavy drinkers. Physical activity was also divided into three groups: low activity, moderate activity and heavy activity.

Table 7.5 Descriptive information regarding the example dataset

	Mean	Standard deviation
Systolic blood pressure (mmHg)	124.5	9.6
BMI	31.2	5.6
Age (years)	61.8	9.3
	Percentage	
Smoking (yes/no)	34.2%/65.8%	
Gender (females/males)	49.9%/50.1%	
Physical activity		
Low	48.5%	
Moderate	31.5%	
Heavy	20.0%	
Alcohol consumption		
Non-drinker	26.1%	
Moderate drinker	38.8%	
Heavy drinker	35.1%	

Furthermore, because the subjects were living in different neighbourhoods an adjustment has to be made for neighbourhood. Table 7.5 shows the descriptive information regarding the dataset used in this example.

The most simple strategy to build a mixed prediction model is comparable to the building of a regular prediction model. The only difference is the fact that (if necessary) a random intercept is added to the prediction model to adjust for the correlated observations within certain groups. A backward or forward selection procedure can be used to get the final prediction model. When a backward selection procedure is used in the present example, the first step is to perform a mixed model analysis with all possible predictor variables in the model and with a random intercept on neighbourhood level. Output 7.14 shows the result of that analysis.

From the first part of Output 7.14, it can be seen that there are 441 observations clustered within 12 neighbourhoods. A random intercept on neighbourhood level is necessary, because the likelihood ratio test (comparing the model with and without a random intercept) given in the last line of the output gives a highly significant p-value. In the fixed part of the model, the regression coefficients, p-values and 95% CIs are given for the potential predictors. When using a backward selection procedure, the

Output 7.14 Result of a linear mixed model analysis to predict systolic blood pressure with all possible predictor variables and with a random intercept on neighbourhood level

```
Mixed-effects ML regression                 Number of obs     =        441
Group variable: neighbourhood               Number of groups  =         12

                                            Obs per group:
                                                        min =         36
                                                        avg =       36.8
                                                        max =         39

                                            Wald chi2(8)      =     392.17
Log likelihood = -1378.1199                 Prob > chi2       =     0.0000

------------------------------------------------------------------------------
    systolic |    Coef.    Std. Err.      z     P>|z|    [95% Conf. Interval]
-------------+----------------------------------------------------------------
         age |  .5213647    .0477432    10.92   0.000    .4277896    .6149397
         bmi |   .507161    .1104761     4.59   0.000    .2906318    .7236902
             |
    activity |
  moderate a.. | -.0284591   .6315857    -0.05   0.964   -1.266344    1.209426
  heavy acti.. | -2.585369   .8272933    -3.13   0.002   -4.206834   -.9639042
             |
     smoking |  -3.650654   1.459801    -2.50   0.012   -6.511812   -.7894973
      gender |  -.3209677   .8699243    -0,37   0.712   -2.025988    1.384053
             |
     alcohol |
  moderate d.. |  1.448811   1.346302     1.08   0.282   -1.189892    4.087514
  heavy drin.. |  1.779286   .8334615     2.13   0.033    .1457314    3.41284
             |
       _cons |  77.24381   3.554645    21.73   0.000    70.27683    84.21079
------------------------------------------------------------------------------


------------------------------------------------------------------------------
  Random-effects Parameters  |   Estimate   Std. Err.    [95% Conf. Interval]
-----------------------------+------------------------------------------------
neighbourh~d: Identity       |
                var(_cons)   |   29.93114   12.63833     13.08295    68.47634
-----------------------------+------------------------------------------------
               var(Residual) |   27.41203    1.87214     23.97768    31.33828
------------------------------------------------------------------------------
LR test vs. linear model: chibar2(01) = 225.15       Prob >= chibar2 = 0.0000
```

first step in the modelling is to take the variable with the highest p-value out of the model. In this example, gender shows the highest p-value, so gender has to be removed from the model. It should be noted that the dummy variable for moderate activity has a higher p-value then gender, but because the dummy variable is part of the predictor physical activity, and the p-value for the dummy variable for heavy activity is very low, activity stays in the model. Output 7.15 shows the result of a mixed model analysis to predict systolic blood pressure without gender as one of the possible predictors.

From the fixed part of the model presented in Output 7.15, it can be seen that all possible predictor variables have significant p-values, so none of the variables can be removed from the model. Output 7.15, therefore, shows the

Output 7.15 Result of a linear mixed model analysis to predict systolic blood pressure with all possible predictor variables, without gender and with a random intercept on neighbourhood level

```
Mixed-effects ML regression                    Number of obs    =         441
Group variable: neighbourhood                  Number of groups =          12

                                               Obs per group:
                                                            min =          36
                                                            avg =        36.8
                                                            max =          39

                                               Wald chi2(7)     =      391.92
Log likelihood = -1378.188                     Prob > chi2      =      0.0000

------------------------------------------------------------------------------
    systolic |     Coef.    Std. Err.      z    P>|z|    [95% Conf. Interval]
-------------+----------------------------------------------------------------
         age |   .5087591   .0333507    15.25   0.000    .4433929    .5741252
         bmi |   .5214324   .1034865     5.04   0.000    .3186025    .7242623
             |
    activity |
  moderate a..|  -.0494987   .6291008    -0.08   0.937   -1.282514    1.183516
 heavy acti.. |  -2.554391   .8231289    -3.10   0.002   -4.167694   -.9410879
             |
     smoking |  -3.658146   1.459874    -2.51   0.012   -6.519446   -.7968461
             |
     alcohol |
  moderate d..|   1.452325   1.346469     1.08   0.281   -1.186706    4.091356
 heavy drin.. |   1.786516   .8333569     2.14   0.032    .153167     3.419866
             |
       _cons |  77.41506   3.525056    21.96   0.000    70.50608    84.32404
------------------------------------------------------------------------------


------------------------------------------------------------------------------
  Random-effects Parameters  |   Estimate   Std. Err.     [95% Conf. Interval]
-----------------------------+------------------------------------------------
neighbourh~d: Identity       |
                  var(_cons) |   29.95848   12.64952     13.09522    68.53728
-----------------------------+------------------------------------------------
                var(Residual)|   27.42004   1.872687     23.98469    31.34743
------------------------------------------------------------------------------
LR test vs. linear model: chibar2(01) = 225.25       Prob >= chibar2 = 0.0000
```

final prediction model to predict systolic blood pressure, taking into account the clustering of the data within the neighbourhood.

A different, slightly more complicated, modelling strategy starts with adding all potential predictor variables to the model. The next step is to evaluate whether or not a random intercept must be allowed. If a random intercept is necessary, the full model with a random intercept is the new starting point. In this full model, for each of the predictor variables, the importance must be evaluated for the situation with and the situation without a random slope for that particular variable. When this has been done for all predictor variables in the model, the variable with the lowest *p*-value can be deleted. Step by step this procedure must be repeated until a certain predefined end-point is reached. Again, this end-point is usually

Output 7.16 Result of a linear mixed model analysis to predict systolic blood pressure with all relevant predictor variables and with a random intercept and random slope for age on neighbourhood level

```
Mixed-effects ML regression                 Number of obs    =       441
Group variable: neighbourhood               Number of groups =        12

                                            Obs per group:
                                                         min =        36
                                                         avg =      36.8
                                                         max =        39

                                            Wald chi2(5)     =    155.90
Log likelihood = -1380.2494                 Prob > chi2      =    0.0000

------------------------------------------------------------------------
    systolic |     Coef.   Std. Err.      z    P>|z|    [95% Conf. Interval]
-------------+----------------------------------------------------------
         age |  .4635239    .050706    9.14   0.000    .3641419    .5629058
         bmi |  .4920706   .1044983    4.71   0.000    .2872576    .6968836
     smoking | -2.823149   1.467675   -1.92   0.054    -5.69974    .0534413
             |
     alcohol |
  moderate d..|  .7278886   1.350689    0.54   0.590   -1.919413    3.37519
  heavy drin..|  1.814655   .8376155    2.17   0.030    .1729586    3.456351
             |
       _cons |  80.60131   4.386772   18.37   0.000     72.0034    89.19922
------------------------------------------------------------------------


------------------------------------------------------------------------
  Random-effects Parameters  |   Estimate   Std. Err.   [95% Conf. Interval]
-----------------------------+------------------------------------------
neighbourh~d: Unstructured   |
                   var(age)  |  .0198461   .0135742     .0051937    .0758359
                 var(_cons)  |  113.0164   68.57732     34.40646    371.2298
           cov(age,_cons)    | -1.295247   .9245687    -3.107368    .5168747
-----------------------------+------------------------------------------
              var(Residual)  |   26.8767   1.866962     23.45568    30.79667
------------------------------------------------------------------------
LR test vs. linear model: chi2(3) = 221.35          Prob > chi2 = 0.0000
```

reached when all independent variables in the model are significant, but sometimes a somewhat less restrictive end-point is used. When the procedure described above has been followed in the example dataset and a cut-off value of $p < 0.10$ is used, the model as shown in Output 7.16 is found to be the best and most simple model to predict systolic blood pressure.

From Output 7.16 it can be seen that the best and most simple model to predict systolic blood pressure consists of age, BMI, smoking and alcohol consumption. It can further be seen that for age a random slope on neighbourhood level is added to the model. It is interesting to compare the result of this modelling procedure with the result of the more simple strategy with only a random intercept, which was shown in Output 7.15. Table 7.6 summarises the results.

Table 7.6 Regression coefficients and standard errors (between brackets) derived from different models in order to predict systolic blood pressure

	Only random intercept	Random intercept and random slopes
Age	0.51 (0.03)	0.46 (0.05)
BMI	0.52 (0.10)	0.49 (0.10)
Smoking	−3.66 (1.46)	−2.82 (1.47)
Gender		
Physical activity		
Moderate	−0.05 (0.63)	
High	−2.55 (0.82)	
Alcohol consumption		
Moderate	1.45 (1.35)	0.73 (1.35)
Heavy	1.78 (0.83)	1.81 (0.84)

From Table 7.6 it can be seen that not only is the magnitude of the regression coefficients different for the different modelling strategies but that the variable physical activity is also present in the model based on the simple modelling strategy but not in the model with the more complicated strategy.

It should (again) be realised that the modelling strategies described in this section are examples of possible modelling strategies, and that there are other (maybe even better) modelling strategies available. Important, however, is the fact that the result of a final prediction or prognostic model (highly) depends on the modelling strategy that is chosen.

In the strategies to build a prediction or prognostic model, no interaction terms were included. Although, theoretically, interaction terms can be part of the final prediction or prognostic model, in practice this is hardly ever done. In most practical situations, it is decided a priori (e.g. based on biological plausibility) that stratified prediction or prognostic models are going to be built. For instance, it can be decided (a priori) that separate prediction or prognostic models are going to be constructed for males and females.

7.3 Prediction and Validation

Based on the final prediction model, the outcome variable can be predicted by the values of the regression coefficients and values of the variables in the model for a particular subject. When a prediction model includes random coefficients, these random coefficients can also be used to predict the outcome variable. Because this is a very interesting feature of mixed model analysis, Chapter 8 will deal with this issue.

It is common sense that after the building of a prediction model, the model must be validated. The best way to do this is an external validation, i.e. the model is used in another comparable dataset to evaluate the performance of the model in the other dataset. Because other comparable datasets are often not available, internal validation is performed, for instance, by calculating the amount of explained variance, the C-statistic, etc. Basically, the internal validation of a prediction model made with mixed model analysis is not different from the internal validation procedures for standard prediction models. See, for details, Steyerberg (2009).

7.4 Comments

In the examples in this chapter, a continuous outcome variable was used. However, dealing with confounding and effect modification as well as the building of association and prediction or prognostic models is exactly the same for dichotomous, categorical or count outcome variables as well as for survival data.

8

Predictions Based on Mixed Model Analysis

8.1 Introduction

Multivariable modelling was discussed in Chapter 7, which included both association models and prediction (or prognostic) models. It was also mentioned that predictions based on a mixed model analysis can include only the regression coefficients, which is basically the same as predictions based on standard multivariable modelling. However, a special feature of mixed model analysis is that it is also possible to include the random coefficients in the prediction. This feature is increasingly popular in prediction modelling, and it is therefore worthwhile discussing this feature in more detail.

8.2 Shrinkage

Let us go back to the example dataset used to explain differences between groups (see Chapter 6). In that dataset the outcome variable was the continuous variable health which was clustered within 28 neighbourhoods. The starting point of the analysis, aiming to explain health differences between neighbourhoods, was a mixed model analysis with a random intercept but without any independent variables. Output 8.1 shows again the result of this analysis.

In Output 8.1 the value of the intercept (11.97488) reflects the average health in the study population, while the random intercept variance (1.356431) reflects the variance in health between neighbourhoods around this average value. When the outcome variable health is predicted by the fixed coefficients, every subject will have the average value (i.e. the

Output 8.1 Result of a linear (intercept-only) mixed model to explain health with a random intercept on neighbourhood level

```
Mixed-effects ML regression                    Number of obs      =          508
Group variable: neighbourhood                  Number of groups   =           28

                                               Obs per group:
                                                              min =            3
                                                              avg =         18.1
                                                              max =           59

                                               Wald chi2(0)       =            .
Log likelihood = -1407.8299                    Prob > chi2        =            .
```

health	Coef.	Std. Err.	z	P>|z|	[95% Conf. Interval]	
_cons	11.97488	.2897764	41.32	0.000	11.40693	12.54283

Random-effects Parameters	Estimate	Std. Err.	[95% Conf. Interval]	
neighbourh~d: Identity				
var(_cons)	1.356431	.5776621	.5887043	3.125346
var(Residual)	14.20534	.9127292	12.52448	16.11178

```
LR test vs. linear model: chibar2(01) = 26.95         Prob >= chibar2 = 0.0000
```

intercept) as predicted value, which is not very interesting. However, within a mixed model setting, the outcome can also be predicted not only by using the (fixed) regression coefficients as well by using the random intercept variance. By using the random intercept variance, different health values are predicted for the different neighbourhoods.

As has been mentioned in Chapter 2, where the basic principles behind mixed model analysis were discussed, the random intercept variance is based on a normal distribution drawn over the separate intercepts for the different neighbourhoods. This normal distribution over the intercepts is now used to get specific intercepts for the different neighbourhoods, which are used in the prediction. Figure 8.1 shows the predicted values for each neighbourhood using the random intercept variance to obtain the predicted value.

It is important to note that the predicted value for each neighbourhood is not equal to the observed average health for that particular neighbourhood.

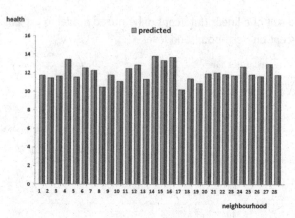

Figure 8.1   Predicted values for each neighbourhood taking into account the random intercept variance.

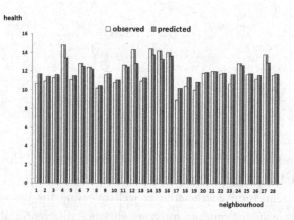

Figure 8.2   Predicted values for each neighbourhood taking into account the random intercept variance compared to the observed values.

This can be seen when the observed average health values are shown next to the predicted values (see Figure 8.2).

From Figure 8.2 it can be seen that for some of the neighbourhoods the predicted health value is higher than the observed value, while for other neighbourhoods the predicted health value is lower than the observed value. In fact, looking at the descriptive information regarding observed and predicted health, it can be seen that the average of the predicted values is equal to the observed average but that the standard deviation of the

Table 8.1 Descriptive information regarding the observed and predicted health values

	Mean	SD	Minimum	Maximum
Observed health	11.98	1.51	8.93	14.80
Predicted health	11.98	1.06	10.18	13.76

SD = Standard deviation.

predicted values is much lower and that the range of predicted health values is much smaller (see Table 8.1).

Looking more carefully to the observed and predicted health values of the different neighbourhoods, it can be seen that for neighbourhoods with a relatively high observed health value (i.e. an observed health value above the overall mean), the predicted value is a bit lower, and for neighbourhoods with a relatively low observed health value (i.e. an observed health value below the overall mean), the predicted value is a bit higher. This phenomenon is known as shrinkage to the mean. Besides that, the amount of shrinkage is not the same for every neighbourhood. In fact, the amount of shrinkage depends on the number of observations in that particular neighbourhood. For neigh-bourhoods with a higher number of observations, the amount of shrinkage is less strong, while for neighbourhoods with a lower number of observations the amount of shrinkage is stronger. Looking at the observed values, pre-dicted values and the number of observations within a neighbourhood, it can be seen that neighbourhood number 12 in the example dataset, for instance, has only six observations; the observed average health value equals 14.33, while the predicted value equals 12.83, i.e. a difference of 1.5. Neighbourhood 14, on the other hand, has 28 observations, an observed health value of 14.43 and a predicted health value of 13.76, i.e. a difference of only 0.67. Table 8.2 shows the observed health values, predicted health values and the number of observations in all neighbourhoods.

From Table 8.2 it can be seen that for neighbourhoods with an observed health value below the overall mean the predicted value is higher than the observed value and that the difference between the two depends on the number of observations within the neighbourhood. The same conclusion, but the other way round, holds for the neighbourhoods with observed health values above the overall mean.

Table 8.2 Observed health, predicted health and number of observations (*N*) for each neighbourhood

Neighbourhood	Observed value	Predicted value	N
1	10.67	11.69	3
2	10.92	11.41	12
3	11.30	11.60	10
4	14.80	13.40	10
5	11.09	11.50	11
6	12.80	12.48	16
7	12.40	12.23	15
8	10.17	10.44	59
9	11.60	11.73	20
10	10.78	11.05	36
11	12.64	12.44	25
12	14.33	12.83	6
13	10.95	11.30	20
14	14.42	13.76	28
15	14.19	13.31	16
16	14.02	13.64	46
17	8.93	10.18	15
18	10.42	11.36	7
19	10.00	10.85	14
21	11.81	11.89	11
22	12.00	11.99	20
23	11.73	11.83	15
24	10.67	11.68	3
51	12.84	12.63	32
52	11.68	11.78	22
53	11.20	11.60	10
55	13.82	12.92	11
56	11.60	11.75	15

The amount of shrinkage can be calculated with Eq. 8.1.

$$\text{shrinkage} = \frac{\sigma_{ij}^2}{\sigma_{ij}^2 + \dfrac{\sigma_e^2}{n_j}} \tag{8.1}$$

Where σ_{ij}^2 = between group variance, σ_e^2 = residual variance and n_j = number of subjects in group j.

8.3 Different Possibilities to Obtain Predicted Values

When a prediction model is created with mixed model analysis, there are basically three possibilities to obtain the predicted values. The first option is a naive prediction in which the possible correlation between the observations within a group is ignored in the model building strategy, so no random intercept nor random slopes are added to the model. This is exactly the same as building a prediction model with a standard regression analysis. For the second option, the possible correlation between the observations within a group is not ignored in the building of the prediction model, so a random intercept and random slopes are considered to be in the model. However, in the prediction only the fixed regression coefficients are used. So, because of the addition of a random intercept and, if necessary, random slopes to the model, only the fixed regression coefficients are changed compared to the naive prediction model, but the random variances are not used in the predictions. In the third option, not only the possible correlations between the observations within a group are used in the building of the prediction model, but the random variances are also used to obtain the predicted values. In the next section the three options will be illustrated with an example.

8.3.1 Example

Let us go back to the example used in Chapter 7 to explain the building of a prediction model within a mixed model setting. The aim of that study was to build a prediction model for systolic blood pressure based on BMI, age, gender, smoking, physical activity and alcohol consumption. In that example a distinction was made between a prediction model including only a random intercept and a prediction model including both a random intercept and (possible) random slopes. Output 8.2 and Output 8.3 again show the final prediction models in both situations.

As has been mentioned before, it is also possible to build a naive prediction model ignoring the correlated observations within a neighbourhood.

Output 8.2 Result of the final linear mixed model analysis to predict systolic blood pressure with a random intercept on neighbourhood level

```
Mixed-effects ML regression                    Number of obs    =       441
Group variable: neighbourhood                  Number of groups =        12

                                               Obs per group:
                                                             min =        36
                                                             avg =      36.8
                                                             max =        39

                                               Wald chi2(7)     =    391.92
Log likelihood =  -1378.188                    Prob > chi2      =    0.0000

------------------------------------------------------------------------------
     systolic |     Coef.   Std. Err.      z    P>|z|     [95% Conf. Interval]
--------------+---------------------------------------------------------------
          age |   .5087591   .0333507    15.25   0.000     .4433929    .5741252
          bmi |   .5214324   .1034865     5.04   0.000     .3186025    .7242623
              |
     activity |
   moderate a..|  -.0494987   .6291008    -0.08   0.937    -1.282514   1.183516
   heavy acti..|  -2.554391   .8231289    -3.10   0.002    -4.167694   -.9410879
              |
     smoking. |  -3.658146   1.459874    -2.51   0.012    -6.519446   -.7968461
              |
      alcohol |
   moderate d..|   1.452325   1.346469     1.08   0.281    -1.186706   4.091356
   heavy drin..|   1.786516   .8333569     2.14   0.032     .153167    3.419866
              |
        _cons |   77.41506   3.525056    21.96   0.000     70.50608   84.32404
------------------------------------------------------------------------------

------------------------------------------------------------------------------
  Random-effects Parameters |   Estimate   Std. Err.     [95% Conf. Interval]
----------------------------+-------------------------------------------------
neighbourh~d: Identity      |
                 var(_cons) |   29.95848   12.64952      13.09522   68.53728
----------------------------+-------------------------------------------------
               var(Residual)|   27.42004   1.872687      23.98469   31.34743
------------------------------------------------------------------------------
LR test vs. linear model: chibar2(01) = 225.25        Prob >= chibar2 = 0.0000
```

Output 8.4 shows the final naive prediction model for systolic blood pressure.

From Output 8.4 it can be seen that the naive prediction model only contains age, BMI and smoking.

Based on the three prediction models and whether the random part of the model is used for prediction or not, five different predicted values can be calculated. Table 8.3 summarises the five different predictions.

Figure 8.3 shows the correlations between the observed systolic blood pressure and the predicted systolic blood pressure from all five methods used to predict systolic blood pressure. Figure 8.4 shows the distribution of the differences between the observed systolic blood pressure and the predicted systolic blood pressure for the five methods to predict systolic blood pressure.

Output 8.3 Result of the final linear mixed model analysis to predict systolic blood pressure with a random intercept and a random slope for age on neighbourhood level

```
Mixed-effects ML regression                     Number of obs      =        441
Group variable: neighbourhood                   Number of groups   =         12

                                                Obs per group:
                                                             min =         36
                                                             avg =       36.8
                                                             max =         39

                                                Wald chi2(5)       =     155.90
Log likelihood = -1380.2494                     Prob > chi2        =     0.0000

------------------------------------------------------------------------------
        systolic |     Coef.   Std. Err.      z    P>|z|    [95% Conf. Interval]
-----------------+------------------------------------------------------------
             age |   .4635239   .050706     9.14   0.000    .3641419    .5629058
             bmi |   .4920706   .1044983    4.71   0.000    .2872576    .6968836
         smoking |  -2.823149   1.467675   -1.92   0.054   -5.69974    .0534413
                 |
         alcohol |
moderate drinker |   .7278886   1.350689    0.54   0.590   -1.919413    3.37519
   heavy drinker |   1.814655   .8376155    2.17   0.030    .1729586    3.456351
                 |
           _cons |   80.60131   4.386772   18.37   0.000    72.0034     89.19922
------------------------------------------------------------------------------

------------------------------------------------------------------------------
  Random-effects Parameters |   Estimate   Std. Err.    [95% Conf. Interval]
----------------------------+-------------------------------------------------
neighbourh~d: Unstructured  |
                 var(age)   |   .0198461   .0135742     .0051937    .0758359
                var(_cons)  |   113.0164   68.57732     34.40646    371.2298
            cov(age,_cons)  |  -1.295247   .9245687    -3.107368    .5168747
----------------------------+-------------------------------------------------
             var(Residual)  |   26.8767    1.866962     23.45568    30.79667
------------------------------------------------------------------------------
LR test vs. linear model: chi2(3) = 221.35          Prob > chi2 = 0.0000
```

Output 8.4 Result of the final naive linear mixed model analysis to predict systolic blood pressure without adjusting for neighbourhood

```
Mixed-effects ML regression                     Number of obs      =        441

                                                Wald chi2(3)       =     352.28
Log likelihood = -1491.1377                     Prob > chi2        =     0.0000

------------------------------------------------------------------------------
        systolic |     Coef.   Std. Err.      z    P>|z|    [95% Conf. Interval]
-----------------+------------------------------------------------------------
             age |   .448969    .0371198   12.10   0.000    .3762155    .5217224
             bmi |   .9853396   .1055933    9.33   0.000    .7783805    1.192299
         smoking |  -3.504123   1.237682   -2.83   0.005   -5.929936   -1.078311
           _cons |   67.2015    3.445057   19.51   0.000    60.44931    73.95368
------------------------------------------------------------------------------

------------------------------------------------------------------------------
  Random-effects Parameters |   Estimate   Std. Err.    [95% Conf. Interval]
----------------------------+-------------------------------------------------
             var(Residual)  |   50.63546   3.409969     44.37433    57.78001
------------------------------------------------------------------------------
```

Table 8.3 Five different possibilities to predict systolic blood pressure

Analysis	Predictions
Naive analysis (Output 8.4)	Only based on the fixed regression coefficients (1)
Random intercept only (Output 8.2)	Only based on the fixed regression coefficients (2)
	Based on both fixed and random coefficients (3)
Random intercept and random slope (Output 8.3)	Only based on the fixed regression coefficients (4)
	Based on both fixed and random coefficients (5)

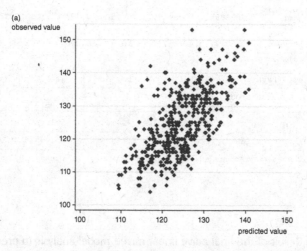

Figure 8.3   (a) Method 1: Naive analysis and predictions only based on fixed regression coefficients. (b) Method 2: Analysis with only a random intercept and predictions only based on fixed regression coefficients. (c) Method 3: Analysis with only a random intercept and predictions only based on both fixed regression coefficients and random variances. (d) Method 4: Analysis with a random intercept and random slope(s) and predictions only based on fixed regression coefficients. (e) Method 5: Analysis with a random intercept and random slope(s) and predictions based on both fixed regression coefficients and random variances.

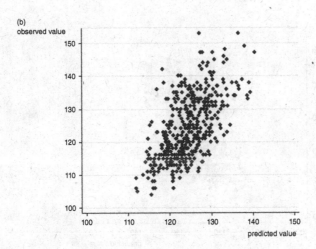

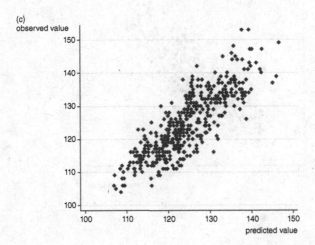

Figure 8.3 (*cont.*)

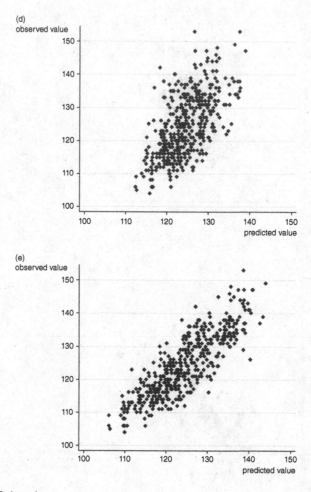

Figure 8.3 (*cont.*)

From the figures with the correlations between the observed and pre-dicted blood pressure values and the figures with the distribution of the differences between the observed and predicted blood pressure values, it can be seen that the predictions using the random coefficients (Methods 3 and 5) are much better than the predictions based on only the fixed regression coefficients. Using only a random intercept for prediction did not differ much from the predictions using both a random intercept and random slopes.

8.4 Comments

Although, in general, the predictions using both the fixed regression coefficients and the random variances are closer to the observed values than the predictions using only the fixed regression coefficients, the use of random variances in the prediction is sometimes criticised by its problematic use in real-life practice. Regarding the example dataset with

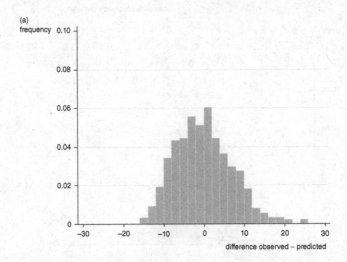

Figure 8.4 (a) Method 1: Naive analysis and predictions only based on fixed regression coefficients. (b) Method 2: Analysis with only a random intercept and predictions only based on fixed regression coefficients. (c) Method 3: Analysis with only a random intercept and predictions only based on both fixed regression coefficients and random variances. (d) Method 4: Analysis with a random intercept and random slope(s) and predictions only based on fixed regression coefficients. (e) Method 5: Analysis with a random intercept and random slope(s) and predictions based on both fixed regression coefficients and random variances.

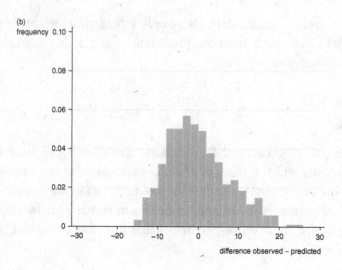

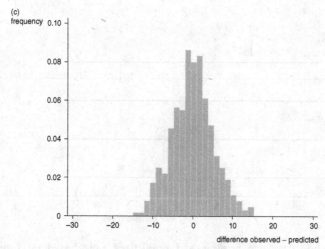

Figure 8.4 (*cont.*)

subjects living in different neighbourhoods: the predictions based on both fixed regression coefficients and random variances can only be used in a proper way for a subject from one of the neighbourhoods that were included in the study from which the prediction model is derived. The predictions for subjects that are living in other neighbourhoods

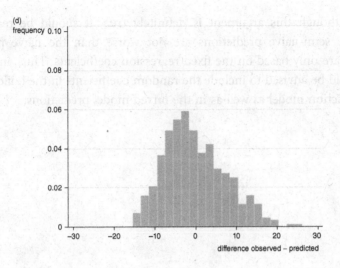

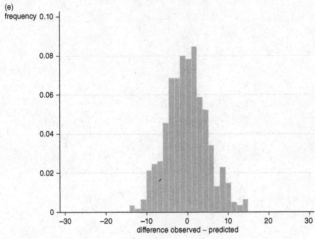

Figure 8.4 (*cont.*)

cannot be done in a proper way, because the random coefficients for that particular neighbourhood are not available. For subjects from other neighbourhoods the prediction can, therefore, only be based on the fixed regression coefficients, assuming that the subjects are living in a sort of average neighbourhood.

Although this argument is definitely true, it should be realised that these semi-naive predictions are not worse than the naive predictions that are only based on the fixed regression coefficients. Thus, in general it should be advised to include the random coefficients in the building of the prediction model as well as in the mixed model predictions.

9

Mixed Model Analysis in Longitudinal Studies

9.1 Introduction

In the earlier chapters it was explained that mixed model analysis is suitable for the analysis of correlated data. Examples were used in which subjects were clustered within neighbourhoods or subjects were clustered within GPs. The fact that observations are correlated is probably most pronounced in longitudinal studies in which repeated observations are made within the subject. It is obvious that these observations are highly correlated. Therefore, the whole theory of mixed model analysis, as described in the earlier chapters, can also be applied to longitudinal data. With longitudinal data the repeated observations are clustered within the subjects (see Figure 9.1).

Figure 9.1 illustrates a two-level structure, i.e. the observations are the lowest level while the subjects are the highest level. This is different from all the examples that have been described before in which the subjects were always the lowest level. It is of course also possible that the subjects are clustered within neighbourhoods, as was the situation in the earlier chapters. This indicates a three-level structure, i.e. the observations are clustered within the subjects and the subjects are clustered within the neighbourhoods (see Figure 9.2).

9.2 Longitudinal Studies

Longitudinal studies are characterised by the fact that the outcome variable is repeatedly measured over time. Table 9.1 shows an example of a typical longitudinal dataset.

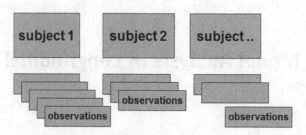

Figure 9.1 Two-level longitudinal mixed model structure; observations are clustered within subjects.

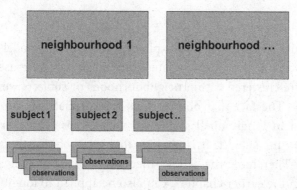

Figure 9.2 Three-level longitudinal mixed model structure; observations are clustered within subjects and subjects are clustered within neighbourhoods.

From Table 9.1 it can be seen that all subjects are measured four times, and that the outcome variable is continuous. There are two independent variables, one time-dependent continuous variable and one time-independent dichotomous variable. Furthermore, there is a variable called time that consists of the observation number for each subject. It should be noted that this dataset has a long data structure, which means that there is one record for each observation. In contrast with the long data structure, there is also a broad data structure in which there is one record for each subject (in a broad data structure the repeated observations are usually referred to as Y_{t1}, Y_{t2}, Y_{t3}, etc.). However, a long data structure is necessary for a mixed model longitudinal data analysis.

Suppose that the aim of the study is to investigate the longitudinal relationship between the time-dependent determinant X and the outcome

Table 9.1 Hypothetical example of a typical longitudinal dataset

Subject	Outcome variable Y	Time-dependent determinant X_1	Time-independent determinant X_2	Time
1	3.5	2.4	1	1
1	3.7	4.3	1	2
1	4.2	4.5	1	3
1	4.5	5.1	1	4
2	1.4	2.8	0	1
2	1.6	2.9	0	2
2	1.7	3.0	0	3
2	1.8	2.7	0	4
...				
...				
N	5.6	5.0	0	1
N	5.6	5.1	0	2
N	5.7	7.5	0	3
N	5.8	6.3	0	4

variable Y. Ignoring the fact that the observations are clustered within the subjects, a standard linear regression analysis can be applied (Eq. 9.1).

$$Y = \beta_0 + \beta_1 X + \varepsilon \tag{9.1}$$

where Y = outcome variable, β_0 = intercept, β_1 = regression coefficient for X, X = time-dependent independent variable and ε = error/residual.

There are probably very few researchers who would perform a standard linear regression analysis on longitudinal data. Everybody is aware of the fact that something different should be done, because the observations within one subject are highly correlated. To cope with this (comparable to the situation in which observations of subjects are clustered within neighbourhoods), an adjustment can be made for subject. This can be done, for instance, by adding the subject number to the model (Eq. 9.2).

$$Y = \beta_0 + \beta_1 X_1 + \beta_2 \text{subject} + \varepsilon \tag{9.2}$$

where: β_2 = regression coefficient for the subject variable.

However, performing a linear regression analysis according to Eq. 9.2 is not correct because it assumes a linear relationship between the subject number and the outcome variable Y; i.e. the regression coefficient for the subject number reflects the difference in outcome Y between subject number 2 and subject number 1, but also the difference in outcome variable Y between subject number 3 and subject number 2, and so on.

In fact, the subject number is not a continuous or discrete variable, it is a categorical (i.e. nominal) variable that must be represented by dummy variables (Eq. 9.3).

$$Y = \beta_0 + \beta_1 X_1 + \beta_2 \text{subject}_1 + \beta_3 \text{subject}_2 + \ldots + \beta_n \text{subject}_{n-1} + \varepsilon \qquad (9.3)$$

where β_2 = regression coefficient for the dummy variable representing the first subject, subject_1 = dummy variable representing the first subject, β_3 = regression coefficient for the dummy variable representing the second subject, subject_2 = dummy variable representing the second subject, subject_{n-1} = dummy variable representing the $n - 1$th subject, etc., and n = number of subjects.

Because a typical longitudinal study usually consists of a few repeated measurements on many subjects, the number of dummy variables will be huge compared to the total number of observations, and therefore it would be impossible to analyse the data in this way. To deal with this, mixed model analysis, again, provides a very elegant solution. It was already mentioned in Chapter 2 that the adjustment for a particular variable, i.e. subject number, actually means that separate intercepts are estimated for each subject. Comparable to what has been discussed for the adjustment for neighbourhood in Chapter 2 within a longitudinal mixed model analysis, a three-step procedure is followed again. First, separate intercepts are estimated for each subject. Then a normal distribution is drawn over the intercepts and finally the variance is estimated from that normal distribution. This variance is added to the model as a random intercept to adjust for the subject. So, instead of many regression coefficients for all dummy variables (representing each subject), only one variance parameter is estimated.

In line with this, it can also be hypothesised that not only the intercepts differ between the subjects but the relationship between X and Y differs too.

In standard linear regression analysis this can be analysed by adding the interaction between X and subject to the regression equation (Eq. 9.4).

$$Y = \beta_0 + \beta_1 X + \beta_2 \text{subject} + \beta_3 \text{subject} \times X + \varepsilon \tag{9.4}$$

where β_3 = regression coefficient for the interaction between the subject variable and the time-dependent determinant X.

Just as for the adjustment, the subject number cannot be treated as a continuous or discrete variable. Because the subject number is a categorical variable which must be represented by dummy variables, the interaction terms should also be made for all dummy variables (Eq. 9.5).

$$Y = \beta_0 + \beta_1 X + \beta_2 \text{subject}_1 + \beta_3 \text{subject}_2 + \dots + \beta_n \text{subject}_{n-1}$$
$$+ \beta_{n+1} \text{subject}_1 \times X + \beta_{n+2} \text{subject}_2 \times X + \dots + \beta_{2n-1} \text{subject}_{n-1} \times X + \varepsilon \tag{9.5}$$

where β_{n+1} = regression coefficient for the interaction between the dummy variable representing the first subject and X, β_{n+2} = regression coefficient for the interaction between the dummy variable representing the second subject and X, β_{2n-1} = regression coefficient for the interaction between the dummy variable representing the $n-1$th subject and X.

Again, given the nature of most longitudinal studies (i.e. a few repeated measurements on many subjects), a large number of regression coefficients must be estimated for all the interaction terms, which is impossible. Again, an elegant solution for this problem is the use of mixed model analysis, in which not all the regression coefficients for each subject are estimated separately, but in which the variance of the regression coefficients is added to the model as a random slope. As for all random coefficients, the variance is based on a normal distribution.

9.2.1 Example

To illustrate the use of mixed model analysis for longitudinal data, an observational longitudinal study is used in which four measurements are performed on 147 subjects. The study aims to analyse the longitudinal relationship between lifestyle and health. Table 9.2 shows descriptive information regarding the example dataset.

Table 9.2 Descriptive information regarding the example dataset

	Mean	Standard deviation	Number of observations
Health	4.30	0.69	588
Lifestyle	3.49	1.40	588

From Table 9.2 it can be seen that there are 588 observations in the example longitudinal dataset. This number of observations is realised by 147 subjects that are measured 4 times. Both variables have 588 observations, so there is no missing data in this example dataset.

The first step in the analysis aiming to analyse the longitudinal relationship between lifestyle and health is to perform a mixed model analysis with a random intercept on subject level. Output 9.1 shows the result of this analysis.

From the first part of Output 9.1 it can be seen that the group variable is subject, that there are 588 observations performed on 147 subjects, and that there are no missing data (4 observations for each subject). In the last line of the output it can be seen that including a random intercept to the model is highly important. The Chi-square value of the likelihood ratio test is extremely high (372.66). The importance of adding a random intercept to the model is also reflected in the magnitude of the ICC, which is 0.72 ($0.320993/(0.320993 + 0.1277738) = 0.715278$). So, there is a very high correlation between the repeated observations within a subject, which is not uncommon in longitudinal studies. In general, the ICC observed in longitudinal mixed model analysis (representing the correlation of repeated observations within subjects) is much higher than the ICC observed in cross-sectional mixed model analysis. In contrast to cross-sectional mixed model analysis, it is not really necessary to evaluate whether a random intercept should be added to the model. In a longitudinal data analysis, a random intercept should always be added to the model, because otherwise the whole idea of a longitudinal study is not taken into account in the analysis. Before going to the interpretation of the regression coefficient, first a random slope for lifestyle on subject level (i.e. the interaction between lifestyle and subject) is added to the model. Output 9.2 shows the result of this analysis.

Output 9.1 Result of a linear mixed model analysis of the longitudinal relationship between lifestyle and health with a random intercept on subject level

```
Mixed-effects ML regression              Number of obs      =        588
Group variable: subject                  Number of groups   =        147

                                         Obs per group:
                                                      min =          4
                                                      avg =        4.0
                                                      max =          4

                                         Wald chi2(1)       =       9.31
Log likelihood = -406.00321              Prob > chi2        =     0.0023

-------------------------------------------------------------------------------
      health |     Coef.   Std. Err.      z    P>|z|     [95% Conf. Interval]
-------------+-----------------------------------------------------------------
   lifestyle |   .070424   .0230807     3.05   0.002     .0251866    .1156613
       _cons |  4.053661   .0942503    43.01   0.000     3.868934    4.238388
-------------------------------------------------------------------------------

-------------------------------------------------------------------------------
  Random-effects Parameters  |   Estimate   Std. Err.     [95% Conf. Interval]
-----------------------------+-------------------------------------------------
subject: Identity            |
                 var(_cons)  |   .320993    .0418752      .2485718    .4145139
-----------------------------+-------------------------------------------------
               var(Residual) |  .1277738    .0086478      .1119005    .1458987
-------------------------------------------------------------------------------
LR test vs. linear model: chibar2(01) = 372.66      Prob >= chibar2 = 0.0000
```

Output 9.2 Result of a linear mixed model analysis of the longitudinal relationship between lifestyle and health with a random intercept and a random slope for lifestyle on subject level

```
Mixed-effects ML regression              Number of obs      =        588
Group variable: subject                  Number of groups   =        147

                                         Obs per group:
                                                      min =          4
                                                      avg =        4.0
                                                      max =          4

                                         Wald chi2(1)       =       8.12
Log likelihood = -405.11858              Prob > chi2        =     0.0044

-------------------------------------------------------------------------------
      health |     Coef.   Std. Err.      z    P>|z|     [95% Conf. Interval]
-------------+-----------------------------------------------------------------
   lifestyle |  .0722621   .0253649     2.85   0.004     .0225477    .1219765
       _cons |  4.046192   .1025121    39.47   0.000     3.845272    4.247112
-------------------------------------------------------------------------------

-------------------------------------------------------------------------------
  Random-effects Parameters  |   Estimate   Std. Err.     [95% Conf. Interval]
-----------------------------+-------------------------------------------------
subject: Unstructured        |
             var(lifest~e)   |  .0101132   .0095825      .0015789    .0647768
                var(_cons)   |  .5110501    .17524        .2609666    1.000788
         cov(lifest~e,_cons) | -.0460515   .039798      -.1240542    .0319513
-----------------------------+-------------------------------------------------
               var(Residual) |  .1234862   .0090491      .1069651     .142559
-------------------------------------------------------------------------------
LR test vs. linear model: chi2(3) = 374.43          Prob > chi2 = 0.0000
```

To evaluate whether a random slope for lifestyle is necessary, a likelihood ratio test can be performed to compare the model with a random slope for lifestyle with the model without a random slope for lifestyle. The $-2\log$ likelihood of the model with only a random intercept was $-2 \times -406.00321 = 812.00642$, while the $-2\log$ likelihood of the model with a random intercept, a random slope for lifestyle and the covariance between the random intercept and random slope was $-2 \times -405.11858 = 810.23716$. The difference between the two equals 1.77, which is not statistically significant on a Chi-square distribution with two degrees of freedom. As always there are two degrees of freedom, because besides the random slope for lifestyle, the covariance between the random intercept and the random slope for lifestyle is estimated as well. So, a random slope for lifestyle is not necessary, and therefore, the regression coefficient of interest can be derived from the model with only a random intercept, which was given in Output 9.1.

The final result of this analysis is that there is a positive longitudinal relationship between lifestyle and health, and the magnitude of that association is 0.070, with a 95% confidence interval (CI) ranging from 0.025 to 0.116 and a p-value of 0.002. The interpretation of the regression coefficient is rather complicated, and is basically twofold: a between-subject interpretation and a within-subject interpretation. The between-subject interpretation is comparable with the standard interpretation of a regression coefficient. When two subjects differ one unit in lifestyle, they differ 0.070 units in health. The within-subject interpretation is typical for a longitudinal study. When lifestyle increases by one unit over a particular time period within a subject, this change is accompanied by an increase of 0.070 units in health of that particular subject. The total regression coefficient of 0.070 is a sort of weighted average of the between-subject relationship and the within-subject relationship. It is possible to disentangle the between-subject and within-subject parts of the relationship by performing a so-called hybrid model analysis (see Section 9.4).

The longitudinal relationship with a continuous outcome variable was analysed in the example. It should be noted that longitudinal mixed model analysis can also be applied to dichotomous, categorical and other outcome variables.

9.3 Hybrid Models to Disentangle Between-Subject and Within-Subject Effects

Hybrid model analysis is used to disentangle the between-subject and within-subject parts of the longitudinal relationship. The between-subject part of the relationship is basically nothing more than the relationship between the mean value of the particular independent variable for each subject and the repeatedly measured outcome variable (Eq. 9.6). To obtain the within-subject part of the relationship, the independent variable can be centred around the mean of the particular subject (Eq. 9.7). The difference between the observations at each time point and the subjects' mean value is known as the deviation score. To obtain both the between-subject and within-subject part of the relationship, a combination of Eqs. 9.6 and 9.7 can be applied (Eq. 9.8).

$$Y = \beta_0 + \beta_b \bar{X} + \varepsilon \tag{9.6}$$

$$Y = \beta_0 + \beta_w (X - \bar{X}) + \varepsilon \tag{9.7}$$

$$Y = \beta_0 + \beta_b \bar{X} + \beta_w (X - \bar{X}) + \varepsilon \tag{9.8}$$

Where Y_{It} = outcome variable measured for subject I at time point t, β_b = regression coefficient for the between-subject part of the relationship, $\bar{X}$ = average value for time-dependent independent variable X, β_w = regression coefficient for the within-subject part of the relationship and X = time-dependent independent variable.

9.3.1 Example

To apply the hybrid model to the example dataset, first the mean value over time for each subject has to be calculated and secondly the deviation score at each time point also has to be calculated. Output 9.3 shows the result of the mixed model analysis with both the individual mean and the deviation score in the model.

From Output 9.3 it can be seen that the between-subject part of the relationship between lifestyle and health is the most important part of the relationship. The regression coefficient for the between-subject part equals

Output 9.3 Result of a linear mixed (hybrid) model analysis of the longitudinal relationship between lifestyle and health with a random intercept on subject level

```
Mixed-effects ML regression                    Number of obs    =       588
Group variable: subject                        Number of groups =       147

                                               Obs per group:
                                                            min =         4
                                                            avg =       4.0
                                                            max =         4

                                               Wald chi2(2)     =     19.07
Log likelihood = -401.41979                    Prob > chi2      =    0.0001

------------------------------------------------------------------------------
      health |    Coef.   Std. Err.      z    P>|z|    [95% Conf. Interval]
-------------+----------------------------------------------------------------
mean_lifest~e |  .1593343  .0367842    4.33   0.000    .0872385    .2314301
dev_lifestyle |   .01624   .029167     0.56   0.578   -.0409262    .0734062
       _cons |  3.743517  .1370168   27.32   0.000    3.474969    4.012064
------------------------------------------------------------------------------


------------------------------------------------------------------------------
  Random-effects Parameters  |   Estimate   Std. Err.    [95% Conf. Interval]
-----------------------------+------------------------------------------------
subject: Identity            |
                var(_cons)  |   .3077503   .0396512     .2390715    .3961587
-----------------------------+------------------------------------------------
               var(Residual) |   .1267816   .0085379     .1111049    .1446702
------------------------------------------------------------------------------
LR test vs. linear model: chibar2(01) = 375.74     Prob >= chibar2 = 0.0000
```

0.1593343 while the regression coefficient of the within-subject part equals 0.01624. It can also be seen from Output 9.3 that the latter is not statistically significant.

The hybrid model can be extended with a random slope, but this can only be done for the within-subject part of the relationship (i.e. the deviation score). The variable reflecting the between-subject part of the relationship (i.e. the subjects' mean score) is not changing over time and therefore is measured on subject level. Because of that, it is not possible to add a random slope for the subjects' mean score to the model. Output 9.4 shows the result of a hybrid model including a random slope for the deviation score.

As with all mixed model analyses, the necessity of the random slope for the deviation score can be evaluated by comparing the -2 log likelihood of the model with only a random intercept with the -2 log likelihood of the model with a random intercept, a random slope for the deviation score and the covariance between the random intercept and random slope. This difference equals 4.78, i.e. $(-2 \times -401.41979) - (-2 \times -399.032) = 802.83958 - 798.064 = 4.77558$, which is not statistically significant on a Chi-square

Output 9.4 Result of a linear mixed (hybrid) model analysis to analyse the longitudinal relationship between lifestyle and health with a random intercept and a random slope for the lifestyle deviation score on subject level

```
Mixed-effects ML regression              Number of obs    =        588
Group variable: subject                  Number of groups =        147

                                         Obs per group:
                                                        min =          4
                                                        avg =        4.0
                                                        max =          4

                                         Wald chi2(2)     =      19.49
Log likelihood =   -399.032              Prob > chi2      =     0.0001

------------------------------------------------------------------------------
      health |      Coef.   Std. Err.      z    P>|z|     [95% Conf. Interval]
-------------+----------------------------------------------------------------
mean_lifest~e |   .1620972   .0367654    4.41   0.000     .0900384     .234156
dev_lifestyle |   .0044306   .0370209    0.12   0.905    -.068129    .0769902
       _cons |   3.733879   .1369554   27.26   0.000     3.465451    4.002307
------------------------------------------------------------------------------

------------------------------------------------------------------------------
  Random-effects Parameters  |   Estimate   Std. Err.     [95% Conf. Interval]
-----------------------------+------------------------------------------------
subject: Unstructured        |
              var(dev_li~e)  |   .0322864   .0197936      .0097091    .1073641
               var(_cons)    |   .3101468   .0396589      .2413921    .3984846
          cov(dev_li~e,_cons)|  -.0086209   .021168      -.0501094    .0328677
-----------------------------+------------------------------------------------
              var(Residual)  |   .1172478   .0088653      .1010983     .135977
------------------------------------------------------------------------------
LR test vs. linear model: chi2(3) = 380.52          Prob > chi2 = 0.0000
```

distribution with two degrees of freedom. So, the final result of this (hybrid) analysis can be derived from the analysis with only a random intercept, as shown in Output 9.3.

Some additional issues regarding the use of hybrid models will be discussed in Section 13.2. For further reading on hybrid models, reference is made to Curren and Bauer (2001) and to Ludtke et al. (2008).

9.4 Growth Curve Analysis

In epidemiological and medical longitudinal studies, mixed model analysis is probably most often applied for the analysis of growth. Growth curve analysis is used to describe the development over time of a particular outcome variable. This specific topic will be explained with the same example dataset that was used in Section 9.3. In the example dataset four measurements were performed for each subject, so basically a third-degree

Output 9.5 Result of a linear mixed model analysis of the linear development of health over time with a random intercept on subject level

```
Mixed-effects ML regression                    Number of obs    =         588
Group variable: subject                        Number of groups =         147

                                               Obs per group:
                                                           min =           4
                                                           avg =         4.0
                                                           max =           4

                                               Wald chi2(1)     =       45.15
Log likelihood = -388.91115                    Prob > chi2      =      0.0000

------------------------------------------------------------------------------
      health |     Coef.   Std. Err.      z    P>|z|    [95% Conf. Interval]
-------------+----------------------------------------------------------------
        time |  -.0840816   .0125133    -6.72   0.000   -.1086072   -.0595561
       _cons |   4.509524   .0598542    75.34   0.000    4.392212    4.626836
------------------------------------------------------------------------------


------------------------------------------------------------------------------
  Random-effects Parameters  |   Estimate   Std. Err.    [95% Conf. Interval]
-----------------------------+------------------------------------------------
subject: Identity            |
                 var(_cons)  |   .3539997   .0446894     .2764051    .4533773
-----------------------------+------------------------------------------------
              var(Residual)  |   .1150879   .0077504     .1008571    .1313265
------------------------------------------------------------------------------
LR test vs. linear model: chibar2(01) = 445.75      Prob >= chibar2 = 0.0000
```

polynomial is the highest-order growth curve that can be modelled. The starting point for a growth curve analysis is a linear development over time. Output 9.5 shows the result of an analysis with only time as an independent variable and with a random intercept on subject level. Again, a random intercept is a conceptual necessity in longitudinal studies, so it is basically not necessary to evaluate this by performing a likelihood ratio test.

From Output 9.5 it can be seen that health is decreasing over time. The regression coefficient for time is −0.0840816, so at each time point health decreases by 0.084 points. It can further be seen that this decrease over time is highly significant. Because there is no missing data, the regression coefficient for time has only a within-subject interpretation, and there is no between-subject part in the estimated relationship between time and health. It should be noted that this is only the case when there is no missing data. When there is missing data, the regression coefficient for time reflects both the within-subject and between-subject part of the relationship between time and health.

The next step in the linear growth curve analysis can be the extension of the model with a random slope for time. Output 9.6 shows the result of this analysis.

Output 9.6 Result of a linear mixed model analysis of the linear development of health over time with a random intercept and a random slope for time on subject level

```
Mixed-effects ML regression               Number of obs     =        588
Group variable: subject                   Number of groups  =        147

                                          Obs per group:
                                                        min =          4
                                                        avg =        4.0
                                                        max =          4

                                          Wald chi2(1)      =      30.91
Log likelihood = -377.18666               Prob > chi2       =     0.0000

------------------------------------------------------------------------------
      health |      Coef.   Std. Err.      z    P>|z|     [95% Conf. Interval]
-------------+----------------------------------------------------------------
        time |  -.0840816    .015124    -5.56   0.000    -.1137242   -.0544391
       _cons |   4.509524   .0597233    75.51   0.000     4.392468    4.626579
------------------------------------------------------------------------------


------------------------------------------------------------------------------
  Random-effects Parameters  |   Estimate   Std. Err.     [95% Conf. Interval]
-----------------------------+------------------------------------------------
subject: Unstructured        |
                 var(time)   |   .0159099   .0041853      .0095005    .0266432
                 var(_cons)  |    .391474   .0621331      .2868162    .5343208
              cov(time,_cons)|  -.0260564   .0129203     -.0513797    -.000733
-----------------------------+------------------------------------------------
              var(Residual)  |   .0885714   .0073052      .0753508    .1041117
------------------------------------------------------------------------------
LR test vs. linear model: chi2(3) = 469.20            Prob > chi2 = 0.0000
```

To evaluate the necessity of the random slope for time, a likelihood ratio test can be performed in which the -2 log likelihood of the model with a random intercept ($-2 \times -388.91115 = 777.8223$) is compared with the -2 log likelihood of the model with a random intercept, a random slope for time and the covariance between the random intercept and random slope ($-2 \times -377.18666 = 754.37332$). The difference between the two -2 log likelihoods equals 23.5, which is highly significant on a Chi-square distribution with two degrees of freedom; again two degrees of freedom because besides the random slope for time, the covariance between the random intercept and the random slope is also estimated.

Up to now a linear development over time has been modelled. However, it is also possible that the development is better described by a second- or third-order polynomial with time. So, the next step in the analysis can be to extend the model with a quadratic time component, i.e. time squared ($time^2$). Output 9.7 shows the result of this analysis.

To evaluate whether or not a second-order polynomial should be used to describe the longitudinal development over time, the p-value for $time^2$ can

Output 9.7 Result of a linear mixed model analysis of the quadratic development of health over time with a random intercept and a random slope for time on subject level

```
Mixed-effects ML regression                 Number of obs    =        588
Group variable: subject                     Number of groups =        147

                                            Obs per group:
                                                         min =          4
                                                         avg =        4.0
                                                         max =          4

                                            Wald chi2(2)     =      31.06
Log likelihood = -377.11138 ·               Prob > chi2      =     0.0000

------------------------------------------------------------------------------
     health |     Coef.    Std. Err.      z    P>|z|     [95% Conf. Interval]
------------+-----------------------------------------------------------------
       time |  -.1078912    .063187    -1.71   0.088    -.2317354    .0159531
      time2 |   .0047619   .0122701     0.39   0.698    -.019287     .0288108
      _cons |   4.533333   .0856198    52.95   0.000     4.365522    4.701145
------------------------------------------------------------------------------


------------------------------------------------------------------------------
  Random-effects Parameters  |   Estimate   Std. Err.     [95% Conf. Interval]
-----------------------------+------------------------------------------------
subject: Unstructured        |
                  var(time)  |   .0159189    .004185 ·     .009509    .0266497
                 var(_cons)  |   .391542    .0621321      .286883    .5343821
             cov(time,_cons) |  -.026079    .0129198    -.0514014   -.0007567
-----------------------------+------------------------------------------------
              var(Residual)  |   .0885261   .0073015     .0753122    .1040584
------------------------------------------------------------------------------
LR test vs. linear model: chi2(3) = 469.32              Prob > chi2 = 0.0000
```

be used. When the relationship with time^2 is not statistically significant, the null-hypothesis is not rejected, and because the null-hypothesis states that the regression coefficient equals zero, a non-significant regression coefficient indicates that (statistically) the regression coefficient equals zero. When the regression coefficient (statistically) equals zero, the second-order polynomial is not better than the first-order polynomial; i.e. a quadratic development over time is not a better than a linear development over time. In Output 9.7 it can be seen that the p-value for time^2 equals 0.689, which is far from significant, so the development over time for health is best described with a linear function.

Due to the non-significant p-value for time^2, it is not expected that a more complicated function over time will better describe the development over time. However, when one wants to evaluate whether a third-order polynomial (an S-shaped curve) better describes the development over time, the same procedure as for the quadratic development over time can be followed. Output 9.8 shows the results of an analysis in which time, time^2 and time^3 are added to the model as independent variables.

Output 9.8 Result of a linear mixed model analysis to analyse the S-shaped development of health over time with a random intercept on subject level

```
Mixed-effects ML regression                Number of obs    =         588
Group variable: subject                    Number of groups =         147

                                           Obs per group:
                                                         min =           4
                                                         avg =         4.0
                                                         max =           4

                                           Wald chi2(3)     =       31.73
Log likelihood = -376.77626                Prob > chi2      =      0.0000
------------------------------------------------------------------------------
   health |      Coef.   Std. Err.      z    P>|z|     [95% Conf. Interval]
----------+-------------------------------------------------------------------
     time |  -.3578231   .3115743    -1.15   0.251    -.9684976    .2528514
    time2 |   .1170068   .1375743     0.85   0.395    -.1526338    .3866474
    time3 |   -.014966   .0182703    -0.82   0.413    -.0507751    .0208431
    _cons |   4.690476   .2100572    22.33   0.000     4.278772    5.102181
------------------------------------------------------------------------------


------------------------------------------------------------------------------
  Random-effects Parameters  |   Estimate   Std. Err.     [95% Conf. Interval]
-----------------------------+------------------------------------------------
subject: Unstructured        |
                 var(time)   |   .0159593   .0041839      .0095469    .0266787
                var(_cons)   |   .3918444   .0621278      .2871797    .5346547
          cov(time,_cons)    |  -.0261798   .0129175     -.0514976   -.0008621
-----------------------------+------------------------------------------------
             var(Residual)   |   .0883245   .0072849      .0751407    .1038214
------------------------------------------------------------------------------
LR test vs. linear model: chi2(3) = 469.87            Prob > chi2 = 0.0000
```

From Output 9.8 it can be seen that the p-value for time^3 is not statistically significant either (p-value = 0.413), so the conclusion of the two analyses is that the development over time for health is best described by a linear function, with both a random intercept and a random slope for time (see Output 9.6). It should be noted that there are different ways to obtain this conclusion. Some authors suggest that one should always start with a model that is as big as possible (i.e. with all possible random variances) and then exclude variances as well as variables with a backward-selection procedure. However, constructing the growth curve in the way that is described in this section provides much more insight into the data. Especially for researchers with (very) little experience in mixed model analysis, the procedure described in this section is highly recommended.

In the example, only possible polynomial functions with time are illustrated. However, it also possible to model other functions with time, such as logistic, logarithmic or exponential functions.

When discrete time points are used in a longitudinal study (as in the present example), time can also be modelled as a categorical variable.

Because modelling time as a categorical variable does not assume a particular mathematical function over time, it makes the analysis a bit more flexible. Four measurements were made of each subject in the example so the categorical time variable must be represented by three dummy variables. The regression coefficients belonging to each of these dummy variables indicate the difference in health between a certain time point and a reference time point, which is usually the first measurement. Output 9.9 shows the results of an analysis in which the development over time for health is modelled with three dummy variables for the categorical time variable. The first measurement is used as a reference category, and in the analysis a random intercept on subject level is added to the model.

From Output 9.9 it can be seen that there are three dummy variables for time. The regression coefficient belonging to the first dummy variable represents the difference in health between the second measurement and the first measurement. This difference is -0.1125646, with a standard error of 0.0395422. The corresponding p-value equals 0.005. The regression

Output 9.9 Result of a linear mixed model analysis of the development of health over time (represented by dummy variables) with a random intercept on subject level

```
Mixed-effects ML regression                    Number of obs     =         588
Group variable: subject                        Number of groups  =         147

                                               Obs per group:
                                                            min =           4
                                                            avg =         4.0
                                                            max =           4

                                               Wald chi2(3)      =       45.85
Log likelihood = -388.59552                    Prob > chi2       =      0.0000

------------------------------------------------------------------------------
     health |      Coef.   Std. Err.      z    P>|z|     [95% Conf. Interval]
------------+-----------------------------------------------------------------
       time |
          2 |  -.1115646   .0395422    -2.82   0.005    -.1890658   -.0340634
          3 |  -.1687075   .0395422    -4.27   0.000    -.2462087   -.0912063
          4 |  -.2612245   .0395422    -6.61   0.000    -.3387257   -.1837233
            |
      _cons |   4.434694   .0564821    78.51   0.000     4.323991    4.545397
------------------------------------------------------------------------------


------------------------------------------------------------------------------
  Random-effects Parameters  |   Estimate   Std. Err.     [95% Conf. Interval]
-----------------------------+------------------------------------------------
subject: Identity            |
                  var(_cons) |   .3540408   .0446893      .2764453    .4534167
-----------------------------+------------------------------------------------
               var(Residual) |   .1149233   .0077393      .1007129    .1311387
------------------------------------------------------------------------------
LR test vs. linear model: chibar2(01) = 446.23         Prob >= chibar2 = 0.0000
```

coefficient for the second dummy variable represents the difference in health between the third measurement and the first measurement. Finally, the regression coefficient belonging to the third dummy variable represents the difference between the fourth measurement and the first measurement.

The next step in the analysis is an extension with random slopes for the three dummy variables. However, a model with random slopes for all three dummy variables did not converge, so the model with only a random intercept will be the final model from which the development over time can be described without assuming a particular mathematical function over time.

It should be noted that the procedure which treats the time variable as categorical is only possible when discrete time points are considered. When the actual time is used for the construction of growth curves, a certain function over time must be modelled.

9.5 Other Methods to Analyse Longitudinal Data

Mixed model analysis is not the only method that is available for the analysis of longitudinal data. Generalised estimating equations (GEE) is another method that is frequently used for the analysis of longitudinal data (Zeger and Liang, 1986, 1992; Lipsitz et al., 1991; Liang and Zeger, 1993; Twisk, 2013). It has already been mentioned in Section 4.4 that the difference between mixed model analysis and GEE analysis is that both methods adjust for the dependency of the observations in different ways. Within mixed model analysis the adjustment is done by modelling the differences between subjects, while within GEE the adjustment is done by directly modelling the correlation within the subject.

The most traditional statistical method to analyse longitudinal data is a generalised linear model (GLM) for repeated measurements. This method is particularly suitable to analyse the development over time in a continuous outcome variable (Twisk, 2013). Because GLM for repeated measurements has some major disadvantages (i.e. no missing data is allowed, it is merely a testing technique) and because the questions answered with a GLM for repeated measurements can also be answered with mixed model analysis and GEE analysis, GLM for repeated measurements is not used much anymore.

Another alternative to analyse longitudinal data is provided by the adjustment for covariance method. This method is comparable to GEE analysis, but different in that it does not model only the within-subject correlation, but also the variance over time (Littel et al., 2000; Twisk, 2013). However, this method is only suitable for the analysis of continuous outcome variables, whereas mixed model analysis and GEE analysis can also be used to analyse dichotomous, categorical and other outcome variables. In order to assess the usefulness of mixed model analysis in longitudinal studies, it is important to describe briefly the similarities and differences in the results of longitudinal data analysis performed with the different methods.

In general, when a continuous outcome variable is analysed, mixed model analysis, GEE analysis and the adjustment for covariance provide more or less the same results, although mixed model analysis is (probably) the most flexible of the three methods. For dichotomous outcome variables, however, the situation is totally different (see also Section 4.4). The regression coefficients of a logistic longitudinal mixed model analysis (i.e. a longitudinal mixed model analysis with a dichotomous outcome variable) are always higher than the regression coefficients obtained from a logistic GEE analysis. This means that the effects estimated with logistic mixed model analysis are more pronounced than those estimated with logistic GEE analysis. However, the standard errors of the regression coefficients are also higher, so the p-values are more or less the same. This difference has been described in Section 4.4 for cross-sectional studies. Equation 4.2 showed the mathematical relationship between the regression coefficient obtained from a logistic mixed model analysis and the regression coefficient obtained from a logistic GEE analysis. This difference was proportional to the differences between the groups (i.e. proportional to the random intercept variance). Because in longitudinal studies the differences between the groups (i.e. the subjects) is much higher than in cross-sectional studies, it is obvious that the difference between the result of a logistic mixed model analysis and a logistic GEE analysis is more pronounced for longitudinal studies (Twisk et al., 2017). In Section 4.4 it has been already mentioned that the effect obtained from a logistic mixed model analysis is an overestimation, and that, therefore, logistic GEE analysis seems to be more appropriate for effect estimation. Besides that, one of the practical problems of logistic longitudinal mixed model analysis is that it seems to be very difficult to estimate the random variances of the regression coefficients, and therefore different estimation procedures lead to different results (see also Sections 4.4 and 13.4.3.4). For a detailed discussion about the differences between mixed model analysis and GEE analysis, reference is made to Neuhaus et al. (1991), Hu et al. (1998), Omar et al. (1999), Crouchly and Davies (2001), Twisk (2004, 2013) and Twisk et al. (2017).

9.6 Comments

9.6.1 Extension of Mixed Model Analysis for Longitudinal Data

The general idea of using mixed model analysis for the analysis of longitudinal data is to adjust for the fact that the observations within subjects are correlated. These correlated observations lead (in general) to correlated errors/residuals, which is the real problem in this kind of regression analysis. In most situations, allowing regression coefficients to differ between subjects (i.e. allowing random regression coefficients) is enough to obtain uncorrelated errors/residuals. However, adding a random intercept and random slope(s) to the model is sometimes not enough to obtain uncorrelated errors/residuals, so an additional adjustment is needed. Therefore, it is possible in some software packages to perform an additional adjustment for the within-subject covariance. It is beyond the scope of this book to discuss this additional adjustment in detail, but basically it is a combination between a mixed model analysis and the adjustment for covariance method. For additional information, reference is made to Pinheiro and Bates (2000), Rabe-Hesketh et al. (2001a, 2001b) and Twisk (2013).

9.6.2 Clustering of Longitudinal Data on a Higher Level

In the examples discussed in this chapter, a two-level structure was considered. Repeated observations were clustered within subjects. It is, of course, also possible that a three-level structure exists, for example, repeated observations are clustered within subjects and subjects are clustered within, for instance, neighbourhoods (see Figure 9.2). It should, however, be noted that when a three-level structure exists in a longitudinal study, GEE analysis and the adjustment for covariance method can no longer be used. Those two techniques are only suitable for a two-level structure. When a three-level structure exists in a longitudinal study, only mixed model analysis can be used.

9.6.3 Missing Data in Longitudinal Studies

One of the biggest problems in longitudinal studies is missing data. There is an enormous amount of literature dealing with this problem (Little and Rubin, 1987; Little, 1995; Schafer, 1997; Allison, 2001), most of which is related to the possible (multiple) imputation of missing data to obtain a complete dataset (Rubin, 1987, 1996; Shih and Quan, 1997; Schafer, 1999). However, when applying mixed model analysis to longitudinal data, there is no need to have a complete dataset. It has been shown that mixed model analysis is very flexible in handling missing data. It has even been shown that applying mixed model analysis to an incomplete dataset is even better than applying (multiple) imputation methods (Twisk and de Vente, 2002; Twisk, 2013; Twisk et al., 2013).

10

Multivariate Mixed Model Analysis

10.1 Introduction

A special feature of mixed model analysis is that it can be used to perform multivariate analysis. Multivariate analysis means that more than one outcome variable is analysed at the same time. In the literature multivariate analyses are often confused with multiple or multivariable analyses, in which the relationship between one outcome variable and more than one independent variable is analysed. Multiple or multivariable modelling was discussed in Chapter 6. Basically, the longitudinal data analysis discussed in Chapter 9 is an example of a multivariate analysis, i.e. the repeated measurements can be seen as multiple outcomes for one individual. Other multivariate analyses are not very common in medical science, but they are (for instance) widely used in psychology. Probably the most frequently applied multivariate statistical technique is the multivariate analysis of variance (MANOVA), in which the average values of more than one continuous outcome variable are compared between groups. MANOVA is a testing technique, and the general idea is that when a significant difference is found between groups the next step is to evaluate which of the outcome variables differs between the groups, or, in other words, which of the outcome variables is related to the group determinant. When no significant difference is observed in the multivariate analysis, this indicates that there is no significant relationship between the group determinant and the separate outcome variables. When multivariate analyses are used in medical or epidemiological studies, it is mostly to analyse the relationship between one or more independent variables and a cluster of outcome variables. In that respect it is comparable with latent variable analysis, in which the cluster of outcome variables are different aspects of a certain (not observable) latent variable. This kind of relationship is often analysed with structural equation modelling (see, for instance, Muthén, 1984; Duncan et al., 1999; Jöreskog and Sörbom, 2001; Skondral and Rabe-Hesketh, 2004). One of the problems with software packages for structural equation modelling is that they are complicated and far from user-friendly. As has been mentioned before, mixed model analysis provides a very elegant alternative to perform a multivariate analysis.

Performing a multivariate mixed model analysis actually means that a level for the different variables must be created below the level of the subject. So, comparable to the situation described in Chapter 9 for longitudinal data analysis, there will be a two-level structure with the different outcome variables as the lower level and the subject as the higher level. Figure 10.1 illustrates this situation in which the outcome variables are clustered within the subject. When the subjects are further clustered (for instance) within neighbourhoods, this will result in a three-level structure (see Figure 10.2).

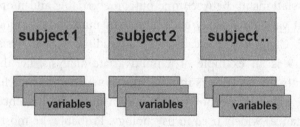

Figure 10.1 Two-level multivariate mixed model structure; variables are clustered within subjects.

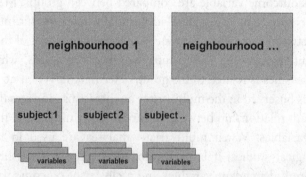

Figure 10.2 Three-level multivariate mixed model structure; variables are clustered within subjects and subjects are clustered within neighbourhoods.

10.2 Example

The application of a multivariate mixed model analysis will be illustrated with an example in which the relationship between two lifestyle indicators, physical activity and alcohol consumption, and well-being is investigated. Well-being is measured with a questionnaire and consists of three domains, physical well-being, psychological well-being and social well-being. The scores on all three domains can range between 0 and 5. Physical activity is expressed in the amount of metabolic equivalents (METs) per week, while alcohol consumption is expressed in the number of glasses of alcohol per day. Table 10.1 shows the descriptive information of the variables used in the example dataset.

Table 10.2 shows the data of the first subject in the dataset. The data structure needed to perform a multivariate mixed model analysis includes a variable domain, which indicates which domain of well-being the value represents, i.e. 1 stands for physical well-being, 2 stands for psychological well-being and 3 stands for social well-being.

Table 10.1 Descriptive information regarding the example dataset

	Mean	Standard deviation
Well-being		
Physical	2.96	1.04
Psychological	3.28	1.05
Social	3.61	1.01
Physical activity (1000 METs/week)	4.88	3.28
Alcohol consumption (glasses/day)	0.86	1.01

Table 10.2 Data of the first subject in the dataset in order to perform a multivariate mixed model analysis

Subject	Well-being	Domain	Alcohol	METs
1	3	1	0.04	2.18
1	4	2	0.04	2.18
1	3	3	0.04	2.18

Output 10.1 Result of a linear mixed model analysis of the relationship between alcohol consumption and overall well-being with a random intercept on subject level

```
Mixed-effects ML regression              Number of obs     =      915
Group variable: subject                  Number of groups  =      305

                                         Obs per group:
                                                        min =        3
                                                        avg =      3.0
                                                        max =        3

                                         Wald chi2(1)      =     7.02
Log likelihood = -1286.7573              Prob > chi2       =   0.0081

------------------------------------------------------------------------
 wellbeing |    Coef.   Std. Err.     z    P>|z|   [95% Conf. Interval]
-----------+------------------------------------------------------------
   alcohol |  .1212413  .0457595    2.65   0.008    .0315543   .2109283
     _cons | 3.167429   .0610402   51.89   0.000   3.047793   3.287066
------------------------------------------------------------------------


------------------------------------------------------------------------
 Random-effects Parameters  |  Estimate   Std. Err.   [95% Conf. Interval]
----------------------------+-------------------------------------------
subject: Identity           |
                 var(_cons) |  .4320627   .0550263    .3366202   .5545663
----------------------------+-------------------------------------------
               var(Residual)|  .684153    .0391745    .6115241   .7654078
------------------------------------------------------------------------
LR test vs. linear model: chibar2(01) = 123.74    Prob >= chibar2 = 0.0000
```

In the first analysis the relationship between alcohol consumption and overall well-being is investigated. In this analysis a random intercept is added to the model to adjust for the correlation of the three well-being measurements within the same subject. This random intercept is a theoretical necessity, comparable to the situation described for longitudinal data analysis in Chapter 9. Output 10.1 shows the result of this analysis.

From Output 10.1 it can be seen that there are 305 individuals in the dataset and that all individuals have three indicators for well-being. Therefore, the total number of observations in the dataset equals 915. The regression coefficient for alcohol consumption (0.1212413) indicates that a one-unit difference in alcohol consumption (i.e. one glass per day) is associated with a 0.12 higher score on overall well-being. Although a likelihood ratio test is not needed to evaluate whether a random intercept should be added to the model since it is a theoretical necessity, the last line of Output 10.1 shows that this likelihood ratio test is highly significant.

From the random part of the regression model the ICC can be calculated. This is done in the usual way by dividing the between-individual

variance by the total variance. In this example, the ICC equals 0.39 (0.43/
(0.43 + 0.68) = 0.39). So, the correlation between the three well-being
domains within the individual is, on average, 0.39. Because alcohol consumption is measured on subject level, it is not possible to add a random
slope for alcohol consumption on subject level to the model. So, the
relationship between alcohol consumption and overall well-being can be
derived from Output 10.1.

In the next step in the analysis, it is interesting to investigate which of the
three domains of well-being is most related to alcohol consumption. To
analyse this, the interaction between domain and alcohol consumption is
added to the model. Output 10.2 shows the result of this analysis.

From Output 10.2 it can be seen that the interaction between domain and
alcohol is statistically significant for the social domain ($p = 0.001$). This

Output 10.2 Results of a linear mixed model analysis to analyse the relationship
between alcohol consumption and three domains of well-being with a random
intercept on subject level

```
Mixed-effects ML regression              Number of obs    =        915
Group variable: subject                  Number of groups =        305

                                         Obs per group:
                                                        min =          3
                                                        avg =        3.0
                                                        max =          3

                                         Wald chi2(5)     =     140.84
Log likelihood = -1226.2648              Prob > chi2      =     0.0000

------------------------------------------------------------------------------
 wellbeing |    Coef.   Std. Err.     z    P>|z|    [95% Conf. Interval]
-----------+------------------------------------------------------------------
    domain |
psycholog~l |  .3402882  .0795848    4.28   0.000    .1843048    .4962717
    social |  .4701563  .0795848    5.91   0.000    .3141729    .6261397
           |
   alcohol |  .080979   .0572751    1.41   0.157   -.0312781    .1932361
           |
   domain#|
 c.alcohol |
psycholog~l | -.075127   .0596617   -1.26   0.208   -.1920617    .0418077
    social |  .1959139  .0596617    3.28   0.001    .0789792    .3128486
           |
      _cons |  2.897281  .0764013   37.92   0.000    2.747537    3.047025
------------------------------------------------------------------------------

------------------------------------------------------------------------------
 Random-effects Parameters  |  Estimate   Std. Err.    [95% Conf. Interval]
-----------------------------+------------------------------------------------
subject: Identity            |
               var(_cons)    |  .4730905  .0545166     .377447    .5929697
-----------------------------+------------------------------------------------
             var(Residual)   |  .5610699  .0321268    .5015074    .6277065
------------------------------------------------------------------------------
LR test vs. linear model: chibar2(01) = 174.86      Prob >= chibar2 = 0.0000
```

significant interaction indicates that the relationship between alcohol consumption and the social domain of well-being is significantly different from the relationship between alcohol consumption and the physical domain (which is the reference category in this analysis). The regression coefficient for alcohol in Output 10.2 (0.080979) indicates the relationship between alcohol consumption and the physical domain of well-being. To obtain the regression coefficient for the two other domains of well-being, the regression coefficient for alcohol has to be added to the regression coefficients for the interaction terms. So, the regression coefficient for the relationship between alcohol consumption and the psychological domain of well-being equals 0.080979 − 0.075127 = 0.005852, and the regression coefficient for the relationship between alcohol consumption and the social domain of well-being equals 0.080979 + 0.1959139 = 0.2768929. To obtain the standard errors of these regression coefficients, the data can be reanalysed with a different domain of well-being as reference category.

Output 10.3 shows the result of the analysis with the psychological domain as the reference category and Output 10.4 shows the result of the same analysis with the social domain as the reference category.

From Output 10.3 it can be seen that the regression coefficient for alcohol in relation with psychological well-being equals 0.005852, and from Output 10.4 it can be seen that the regression coefficient for alcohol in relation with social well-being equals 0.2768929. These regression coefficients were already calculated based on Output 10.2, but from Output 10.3 and Output 10.4, the 95% CI around the regression coefficients and the corresponding p-values can also be derived.

Table 10.3 summarises the results of the analyses performed on the relationship between alcohol consumption and well-being and the different domains of well-being.

From Table 10.3 it can be seen that alcohol consumption is specifically related to the social domain of well-being and less to other two domains. Furthermore, it can be seen that there is almost no relationship between alcohol consumption and the psychological domain of well-being.

In the same way, the relationship between physical activity and (the different domains of) well-being can be investigated. Output 10.5 shows the results of the analysis performed to evaluate the relationship between

Output 10.3 Result of a linear mixed model analysis of the relationship between alcohol consumption and three domains of well-being (with the psychological domain as reference) with a random intercept on subject level

```
Mixed-effects ML regression                    Number of obs      =         915
Group variable: id                             Number of groups   =         305

                                               Obs per group:
                                                             min =           3
                                                             avg =         3.0
                                                             max =           3

                                               Wald chi2(5)       =      140.84
Log likelihood = -1226.2648                    Prob > chi2        =      0.0000
```

wellbeing	Coef.	Std. Err.	z	P>|z|	[95% Conf. Interval]	
domain						
physical	-.3402882	.0795848	-4.28	0.000	-.4962717	-.1843048
social	.1298681	.0795848	1.63	0.103	-.0261153	.2858515
alcohol	.005852	.0572751	0.10	0.919	-.1064051	.1181091
domain#						
c.alcohol						
physical	.075127	.0596617	1.26	0.208	-.0418077	.1920617
social	.2710409	.0596617	4.54	0.000	.1541062	.3879756
_cons	3.237569	.0764013	42.38	0.000	3.087825	3.387313

Random-effects Parameters	Estimate	Std. Err.	[95% Conf. Interval]	
id: Identity				
var(_cons)	.4730905	.0545166	.377447	.5929697
var(Residual)	.5610699	.0321268	.5015074	.6277065

```
LR test vs. linear model: chibar2(01) = 174.86          Prob >= chibar2 = 0.0000
```

physical activity and overall well-being, with a random intercept on subject level.

Output 10.6 shows the result of the multivariate mixed model analysis of the relationship between physical activity and the different domains of well-being, with a random intercept on subject level using the physical domain as reference category.

To obtain the regression coefficient, 95% CI and corresponding p-values for the relationship between physical activity and the other two domains of well-being, the data is reanalysed with different reference categories for well-being. Output 10.7 and Output 10.8 show the result of these analyses and Table 10.4 summarises the results of the analyses.

From Table 10.4 it can be seen that physical activity is mostly related to the physical domain of well-being. The regression coefficient indicates that

Output 10.4 Results of a linear mixed model analysis of the relationship between alcohol consumption and three domains of well-being (with the social domain as reference) with a random intercept on subject level

```
Mixed-effects ML regression                    Number of obs    =        915
Group variable: id                             Number of groups =        305

                                               Obs per group:
                                                            min =          3
                                                            avg =        3.0
                                                            max =          3

                                               Wald chi2(5)     =     140.84
Log likelihood = -1226.2648                    Prob > chi2      =     0.0000

-------------------------------------------------------------------------------
   wellbeing |     Coef.   Std. Err.      z    P>|z|     [95% Conf. Interval]
-------------+-----------------------------------------------------------------
      domain |
    physical |  -.4701563   .0795848    -5.91   0.000    -.6261397   -.3141729
 psycholog~1 |  -.1298681   .0795848    -1.63   0.103    -.2858515    .0261153
             |
     alcohol |   .2768929   .0572751     4.83   0.000     .1646358     .38915
             |
     domain# |
   c.alcohol |
    physical |  -.1959139   .0596617    -3.28   0.001    -.3128486   -.0789792
 psycholog~1 |  -.2710409   .0596617    -4.54   0.000    -.3879756   -.1541062
             |
       _cons |   3.367437   .0764013    44.08   0.000     3.217694    3.517181
-------------------------------------------------------------------------------

-------------------------------------------------------------------------------
  Random-effects Parameters  |   Estimate   Std. Err.    [95% Conf. Interval]
-----------------------------+-------------------------------------------------
id: Identity                 |
               var(_cons)    |   .4730905   .0545166      .377447     .5929697
-----------------------------+-------------------------------------------------
            var(Residual)    |   .5610699   .0321268     .5015074     .6277065
-------------------------------------------------------------------------------
LR test vs. linear model: chibar2(01) = 174.86        Prob >= chibar2 = 0.0000
```

Table 10.3 Summary of the results of (multivariate) mixed model analysis of the relationship between alcohol consumption and (different domains of) well-being

	Coefficient	95% CI	p-value
Overall well-being	0.11	0.04 to 0.19	0.002
Domains			
Physical	0.08	−0.03 to 0.19	0.16
Psychological	0.006	−0.11 to 0.12	0.92
Social	0.28	0.16 to 0.39	<0.001

Output 10.5 Results of a linear mixed model analysis of the relationship between physical activity and well-being with a random intercept on subject level

```
Mixed-effects ML regression                    Number of obs    =        927
Group variable: subject                        Number of groups =        309

                                               Obs per group:
                                                         min =          3
                                                         avg =        3.0
                                                         max =          3

                                               Wald chi2(1)     =       5.55
Log likelihood = -1303.8636                    Prob > chi2      =     0.0185

------------------------------------------------------------------------------
  wellbeing |     Coef.   Std. Err.      z    P>|z|    [95% Conf. Interval]
------------+-----------------------------------------------------------------
   activity |  .0344046   .0146032     2.36   0.018    .0057829    .0630263
      _cons |  3.099093   .0854828    36.25   0.000     2.93155    3.266636
------------------------------------------------------------------------------

------------------------------------------------------------------------------
  Random-effects Parameters  |   Estimate   Std. Err.    [95% Conf. Interval]
-----------------------------+------------------------------------------------
subject: Identity            |
                 var(_cons)  |   .4534559   .0560727     .3558595    .5778187
-----------------------------+------------------------------------------------
               var(Residual) |   .6752966   .0384163     .6040479    .7549492
------------------------------------------------------------------------------
LR test vs. linear model: chibar2(01) = 135.26      Prob >= chibar2 = 0.0000
```

Output 10.6 Result of a linear mixed model analysis of the relationship between physical activity and three domains of well-being with a random intercept on subject level

```
Mixed-effects ML regression                    Number of obs    =        927
Group variable: subject                        Number of groups =        309

                                               Obs per group:
                                                         min =          3
                                                         avg =        3.0
                                                         max =          3

                                               Wald chi2(5)     =     165.84
Log likelihood = -1232.6066                    Prob > chi2      =     0.0000

------------------------------------------------------------------------------
  wellbeing |     Coef.   Std. Err.      z    P>|z|    [95% Conf. Interval]
------------+-----------------------------------------------------------------
     domain |
 psycholog~1 |  .8510122   .1074665     7.92   0.000    .6403817    1.061643
      social |  .9998973   .1074665     9.30   0.000    .7892669    1.210528
             |
    activity |  .0991705   .0180444     5.50   0.000    .0638041    .1345369
             |
    domain#|
  c.activity |
 psycholog~1 | -.1196221   .0183587    -6.52   0.000   -.1556045   -.0836397
      social | -.0746756   .0183587    -4.07   0.000    -.110658   -.0386932
             |
       _cons |  2.482123   .1056266    23.50   0.000    2.275099    2.689148
------------------------------------------------------------------------------

------------------------------------------------------------------------------
  Random-effects Parameters  |   Estimate   Std. Err.    [95% Conf. Interval]
-----------------------------+------------------------------------------------
subject: Identity            |
                 var(_cons)  |   .4998145   .0555299     .4020125    .6214099
-----------------------------+------------------------------------------------
               var(Residual) |   .5362211   .0305046     .4796459    .5994695
------------------------------------------------------------------------------
LR test vs. linear model: chibar2(01) = 198.32      Prob >= chibar2 = 0.0000
```

Output 10.7 Results of a linear mixed model analysis to analyse the relationship between physical activity and three domains of well-being (with the psychological domain as reference) with a random intercept on subject level

```
Mixed-effects ML regression                    Number of obs      =        927
Group variable: subject                        Number of groups   =        309

                                               Obs per group:
                                                            min =          3
                                                            avg =        3.0
                                                            max =          3

                                               Wald chi2(5)       =     165.84
Log likelihood = -1232.6066                    Prob > chi2        =     0.0000

------------------------------------------------------------------------------
  wellbeing |     Coef.   Std. Err.      z    P>|z|     [95% Conf. Interval]
------------+-----------------------------------------------------------------
     domain |
   physical |  -.8510122   .1074665   -7.92   0.000    -1.061643   -.6403817
     social |   .1488851   .1074665    1.39   0.166    -.0617453    .3595155
            |
   activity |  -.0204516   .0180444   -1.13   0.257    -.0558179    .0149148
            |
    domain#|
 c.activity |
   physical |   .1196221   .0183587    6.52   0.000     .0836397    .1556045
     social |   .0449465   .0183587    2.45   0.014     .0089641    .0809289
            |
      _cons |   3.333135   .1056266   31.56   0.000     3.126111    3.54016
------------------------------------------------------------------------------


------------------------------------------------------------------------------
  Random-effects Parameters  |   Estimate   Std. Err.    [95% Conf. Interval]
-----------------------------+------------------------------------------------
subject: Identity            |
                 var(_cons)  |   .4998145   .0555299     .4020125    .6214099
-----------------------------+------------------------------------------------
               var(Residual) |   .5362211   .0305046     .4796459    .5994695
------------------------------------------------------------------------------
LR test vs. linear model: chibar2(01) = 198.32        Prob >= chibar2 = 0.0000
```

a one unit difference in physical activity (1000 METs/week) is associated with a 0.099 higher score on physical well-being.

Because alcohol consumption and physical activity are probably related to each other, it is also possible to analyse both independent variables together in order to obtain the independent relationships between alcohol consumption, physical activity and (several domains of) well-being. Output 10.9, Output 10.10, Output 10.11 and Output 10.12 show the results of these combined multivariate mixed model analyses and Table 10.5 summarises the results. In all analyses a random intercept on subject level is added to the model.

When the results obtained from the univariable multivariate mixed model analyses (Table 10.4) are compared to the results of the multivariable

Output 10.8 Result of a linear mixed model analysis of the relationship between physical activity and three domains of well-being (with the social domain as reference) with a random intercept on subject level

```
Mixed-effects ML regression                    Number of obs     =        927
Group variable: subject                        Number of groups  =        309

                                               Obs per group:
                                                            min =          3
                                                            avg =        3.0
                                                            max =          3

                                               Wald chi2(5)      =     165.84
Log likelihood = -1232.6066                    Prob > chi2       =     0.0000

------------------------------------------------------------------------------
   wellbeing |     Coef.   Std. Err.      z    P>|z|    [95% Conf. Interval]
-------------+----------------------------------------------------------------
      domain |
    physical | -.9998973   .1074665    -9.30   0.000   -1.210528   -.7892669
 psycholog~l | -.1488851   .1074665    -1.39   0.166   -.3595155    .0617453
             |
    activity |  .0244949   .0180444     1.36   0.175   -.0108714    .0598613
             |
      domain#|
  c.activity |
    physical |  .0746756   .0183587     4.07   0.000    .0386932    .110658
 psycholog~l | -.0449465   .0183587    -2.45   0.014   -.0809289   -.0089641
             |
       _cons |  3.482021   .1056266    32.97   0.000    3.274996    3.689045
------------------------------------------------------------------------------


------------------------------------------------------------------------------
  Random-effects Parameters  |   Estimate   Std. Err.     [95% Conf. Interval]
-----------------------------+------------------------------------------------
subject: Identity            |
                 var(_cons)  |   .4998145   .0555299      .4020125    .6214099
-----------------------------+------------------------------------------------
               var(Residual) |   .5362211   .0305046      .4796459    .5994695
------------------------------------------------------------------------------
LR test vs. linear model: chibar2(01) = 198.32      Prob >= chibar2 = 0.0000
```

Output 10.9 Result of a linear mixed model analysis of the relationship between alcohol consumption, physical activity and overall well-being with a random intercept on subject level

```
Mixed-effects ML regression                    Number of obs     =        912
Group variable: subject                        Number of groups  =        304

                                               Obs per group:
                                                            min =          3
                                                            avg =        3.0
                                                            max =          3

                                               Wald chi2(2)      =      15.11
Log likelihood = -1276.6985                    Prob > chi2       =     0.0005

------------------------------------------------------------------------------
   wellbeing |     Coef.   Std. Err.      z    P>|z|    [95% Conf. Interval]
-------------+----------------------------------------------------------------
     alcohol |    .13842   .0457317     3.03   0.002    .0487876    .2280525
    activity |  .0405718   .0144059     2.82   0.005    .0123368    .0688068
       _cons |  2.953371   .0970617    30.43   0.000    2.763134    3.143609
------------------------------------------------------------------------------


------------------------------------------------------------------------------
  Random-effects Parameters  |   Estimate   Std. Err.     [95% Conf. Interval]
-----------------------------+------------------------------------------------
subject: Identity            |
                 var(_cons)  |   .4191851   .0539353      .3257499    .5394203
-----------------------------+------------------------------------------------
               var(Residual) |    .678728   .0389277      .6065632    .7594786
------------------------------------------------------------------------------
LR test vs. linear model: chibar2(01) = 119.94      Prob >= chibar2 = 0.0000
```

Table 10.4 Summary of the results of (multivariate) mixed model analysis of the relationship between physical activity and (different domains of) well-being

	Coefficient	95% CI	p-value
Overall well-being	0.034	0.006 to 0.063	0.018
Domains			
Physical	0.099	0.064 to 0.135	<0.001
Psychological	−0.02	−0.056 to 0.015	0.26
Social	0.024	−0.011 to 0.06	0.18

Output 10.10 Result of a linear mixed model analysis of the relationship between alcohol consumption, physical activity and three domains of well-being (with the physical domain as reference) with a random intercept on subject level

```
Mixed-effects ML regression              Number of obs    =        912
Group variable: subject                  Number of groups =        304

                                         Obs per group:
                                                        min =          3
                                                        avg =        3.0
                                                        max =          3

                                         Wald chi2(8)     =     204.80
Log likelihood = -1194.1518              Prob > chi2      =     0.0000

------------------------------------------------------------------------------
   wellbeing |     Coef.   Std. Err.      z    P>|z|    [95% Conf. Interval]
-------------+----------------------------------------------------------------
      domain |
 psycholog~1 |   1.013142   .122892     8.24   0.000     .7722777    1.254006
      social |   .8314398   .122892     6.77   0.000     .5905759    1.072304
             |
     alcohol |   .1288916   .0566474    2.28   0.023     .0178647    .2399185
             |
     domain# |
   c.alcohol |
 psycholog~1 |  -.1311778   .0579019   -2.27   0.023    -.2446635   -.0176921
      social |   .1597632   .0579019    2.76   0.006     .0462775    .2732489
             |
    activity |   .105951    .0178444    5.94   0.000     .0709766    .1409254
             |
     domain# |
  c.activity |
 psycholog~1 |  -.1275595   .0182396   -6.99   0.000    -.1633084   -.0918105
      social |  -.0685782   .0182396   -3.76   0.000    -.1043271   -.0328292
             |
       _cons |   2.338511   .1202294   19.45   0.000     2.102865    2.574156
------------------------------------------------------------------------------

------------------------------------------------------------------------------
  Random-effects Parameters  |   Estimate   Std. Err.     [95% Conf. Interval]
-----------------------------+------------------------------------------------
subject: Identity            |
                  var(_cons) |   .4729838   .0532772      .3792856     .589829
-----------------------------+------------------------------------------------
                var(Residual)|   .5173323   .029671       .4623276    .5788811
------------------------------------------------------------------------------
LR test vs. linear model: chibar2(01) = 190.97      Prob >= chibar2 = 0.0000
```

Table 10.5 Summary of the results of (multivariate) mixed model analysis of the relationship between physical activity, alcohol consumption and (different domains of) well-being

	Coefficient	95% CI	p-value
Alcohol consumption			
Overall well-being	0.14	0.05 to 0.23	0.002
Domains			
Physical	0.13	0.02 to 0.24	0.023
Psychological	−0.002	−0.11 to 0.11	0.97
Social	0.29	0.18 to 0.4	<0.001
Physical activity			
Overall well-being	0.041	0.012 to 0.069	0.006
Domains			
Physical	0.106	0.071 to 0.141	<0.001
Psychological	−0.022	−0.057 to 0.013	0.23
Social	0.037	0.002 to 0.072	0.04

multivariate mixed model analyses (Table 10.5), it can be seen that the results are not particularly different; although, in general, the regression coefficients are slightly higher in the multivariable analyses. This causes the positive relationship between alcohol consumption and physical well-being to be statistically significant in the multivariable analysis, which also holds for the positive relationship between physical activity and social well-being.

10.3 Comments

Some researchers argue that the result of the overall analysis determines the following steps in the analysis. This argument is based on testing theory and indicates that an analysis relating an independent variable to (in this particular example) the different domains of well-being should only be done when the overall relationship is statistically significant. This is, however, not a good argument to decide whether these analyses should be performed. The decision whether analyses relating the independent variables to the different domains of well-being should be performed must be based on the research question. In this particular example it is highly

Output 10.11 Result of a linear mixed model analysis to analyse the relationship between alcohol consumption, physical activity and three domains of well-being (with the psychological domain as reference) with a random intercept on subject level

```
Mixed-effects ML regression                 Number of obs     =        912
Group variable: subject                     Number of groups  =        304

                                            Obs per group:
                                                         min =          3
                                                         avg =        3.0
                                                         max =          3

                                            Wald chi2(8)      =     204.80
Log likelihood = -1194.1518                 Prob > chi2       =     0.0000
```

wellbeing	Coef.	Std. Err.	z	P>|z|	[95% Conf. Interval]	
domain						
physical	-1.013142	.122892	-8.24	0.000	-1.254006	-.7722777
social	-.1817018	.122892	-1.48	0.139	-.4225658	.0591621
alcohol	-.0022862	.0566474	-0.04	0.968	-.1133131	.1087407
domain#|						
c.alcohol						
physical	.1311778	.0579019	2.27	0.023	.0176921	.2446635
social	.290941	.0579019	5.02	0.000	.1774553	.4044267
activity	-.0216085	.0178444	-1.21	0.226	-.0565829	.013366
domain#|						
c.activity						
physical	.1275595	.0182396	6.99	0.000	.0918105	.1633084
social	.0589813	.0182396	3.23	0.001	.0232324	.0947303
_cons	3.351652	.1202294	27.88	0.000	3.116007	3.587298

Random-effects Parameters	Estimate	Std. Err.	[95% Conf. Interval]	
subject: Identity				
var(_cons)	.4729838	.0532772	.3792856	.589829
var(Residual)	.5173323	.029671	.4623276	.5788811

```
LR test vs. linear model: chibar2(01) = 190.97      Prob >= chibar2 = 0.0000
```

interesting to investigate the relationship between the independent variables and the different domains of well-being, irrespective of the p-value of the overall relationship.

To obtain the relationship between the independent variables and the different domains of well-being it is, of course, also possible to perform stratified analysis for the three domains. However, when the analysis are stratified it is assumed that the analyses are independent of each other. Based on the results of the analyses performed in this chapter, it can be concluded that the assumption of independence definitely does not hold.

Output 10.12 .Result of a linear mixed model analysis to analyse the relationship between alcohol consumption, physical activity and three domains of well-being (with the social domain as reference) with a random intercept on subject level

```
Mixed-effects ML regression                 Number of obs    =       912
Group variable: subject                     Number of groups =       304

                                            Obs per group:
                                                         min =         3
                                                         avg =       3.0
                                                         max =         3

                                            Wald chi2(8)     =    204.80
Log likelihood = -1194.1518                 Prob > chi2      =    0.0000
```

wellbeing	Coef.	Std. Err.	z	P>|z|	[95% Conf. Interval]	
domain						
physical	-.8314398	.122892	-6.77	0.000	-1.072304	-.5905759
psycholog~l	.1817018	.122892	1.48	0.139	-.0591621	.4225658
alcohol	.2886548	.0566474	5.10	0.000	.1776279	.3996817
domain#						
c.alcohol						
physical	-.1597632	.0579019	-2.76	0.006	-.2732489	-.0462775
psycholog~l	-.290941	.0579019	-5.02	0.000	-.4044267	-.1774553
activity	.0373729	.0178444	2.09	0.036	.0023985	.0723473
domain#						
c.activity						
physical	.0685782	.0182396	3.76	0.000	.0328292	.1043271
psycholog~l	-.0589813	.0182396	-3.23	0.001	-.0947303	-.0232324
_cons	3.169951	.1202294	26.37	0.000	2.934305	3.405596

Random-effects Parameters	Estimate	Std. Err.	[95% Conf. Interval]	
subject: Identity				
var(_cons)	.4729838	.0532772	.3792856	.589829
var(Residual)	.5173323	.029671	.4623276	.5788811

```
LR test vs. linear model: chibar2(01) = 190.97          Prob >= chibar2 = 0.0000
```

In this particular example, the scale on which the three domains of well-being were expressed was the same. All scales range between 0 and 5 and, therefore, the same interpretation holds for all three domains. It should be realised that when the scale on which the different domains or the different variables analysed in the multivariate mixed model analysis differ, the interpretation of the multivariate analysis will be difficult. A possible solution for this potential problem is to standardise the values for the different domains or variables used in the multivariate analysis.

Meta-Analysis on Individual Participant Data

11.1 Introduction

Individual participant data (IPD) meta-analysis is a relatively new technique to examine treatment effects by combining individual participant data from multiple trials. IPD meta-analysis uses the same basic approach as any other systematic review and meta-analysis, however, it involves collection of the original data from as many of the relevant trials as can be accessed. IPD meta-analysis is seen as a sort of golden standard in the field of meta-analysis and has several advantages over standard meta-analysis, including increased statistical power to examine predictors and moderators of the intervention effect. Besides that, the advantage of an IPD meta-analysis is that the meta-analysis is not limited to the information provided in the published papers nor is limited by the statistical analysis performed in the papers involved in the meta-analysis. The general idea behind IPD meta-analysis is that effects are estimated based on the participant data instead of that the effects are estimated based on the published effects for each study. Basically there are two possibilities for an IPD meta-analysis: two-stage IPD meta-analysis and one-stage IPD meta-analysis. In a two-stage IPD meta-analysis, the effect of a particular treatment is estimated within each study separately in the first stage, and these effects are combined with each other in a standard meta-analysis in the second stage. In a one-stage IPD meta-analysis, the effect of a particular treatment is estimated directly in the combined dataset that includes data from all studies. The latter implicates that the data is correlated within the study and that mixed model analysis can be used to take into account the clustered observations. So, in this particular implication of mixed model analysis, the individual participant data is clustered within studies (see Figure 11.1).

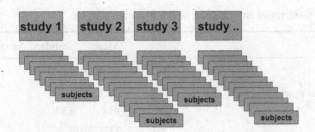

Figure 11.1 Two-level mixed model structure; subjects are clustered within studies.

Basically, a one-stage IPD meta-analysis is nothing more than a two-level mixed model analysis in which the subjects are clustered within studies. So, all the basic principles discussed in Chapter 2 also hold for a one-stage IPD meta-analysis. The next section will illustrate the use of mixed models for a one-stage IPD meta-analysis.

11.2 Example

The example dataset contains data from nine studies investigating the effect of a new treatment aiming to decrease depressive symptoms. Depressive symptoms were measured with the same questionnaire in all studies. As a result of the questionnaire, a continuous outcome variable was created – for which high values indicate more symptoms. Besides the depression measurement after treatment, in all studies the baseline value of the depression score and some other covariates were measured as well. Table 11.1 shows descriptive information regarding the total dataset used in the example.

To perform an IPD meta-analysis, a mixed model analysis is performed with a random intercept on study level to take into account the clustering of the data within the studies. Output 11.1 shows the result of this analysis.

From the last line of Output 11.1 it can be seen that an adjustment for study by adding a random intercept to the model was necessary. The likelihood ratio test revealed a highly significant p-value (<0.001), which is based on a Chi-square value of 28.30 and a Chi-square distribution with one degree of freedom. The ICC in this situation can be calculated by dividing the between-study variance (6.617402) by the total variance (6.617402 + 78.21775) = 0.078. The treatment effect can be derived from

Table 11.1 Descriptive information of the example dataset

	Mean	Standard deviation	N
Depression	16.0	9.9	574
Depression at baseline	25.3	8.1	607
Age	41.0	13.1	607
	Percentage		
Treatment (no/yes)	48.8%/51.2%		607
Gender (females/males)	76.6%/23.4%		607
Education (low/moderate/high)	5.3%/23.4%/71.3%		568
Marital status (married/single/divorced_widowed)	52.9%/68.6%/13.4%		531

Output 11.1 Result of a linear IPD mixed model analysis to determine the effect of a treatment on depression adjusted for baseline differences and with a random intercept on study level

```
Mixed-effects ML regression                    Number of obs      =        574
Group variable: study                          Number of groups   =          9

                                               Obs per group:
                                                             min =         47
                                                             avg =       63.8
                                                             max =         89

                                               Wald chi2(2)       =      87.06
Log likelihood = -2073.9191                    Prob > chi2        =     0.0000

------------------------------------------------------------------------------
 depression |     Coef.   Std. Err.       z    P>|z|    [95% Conf. Interval]
------------+-----------------------------------------------------------------
  treatment | -3.172244   .7424377    -4.27    0.000   -4.627396   -1.717093
 depression0 |  .3869113   .0471819     8.20    0.000    .2944364    .4793861
      _cons |  7.747245   1.568191     4.94    0.000    4.673647    10.82084
------------------------------------------------------------------------------


------------------------------------------------------------------------------
 Random-effects Parameters  |   Estimate   Std. Err.     [95% Conf. Interval]
----------------------------+-------------------------------------------------
study: Identity             |
                 var(_cons) |   6.617402   3.752064     2.177994    20.10566
----------------------------+-------------------------------------------------
              var(Residual) |   78.21775   4.654264     69.60741    87.89318
------------------------------------------------------------------------------
LR test vs. linear model: chibar2(01) = 28.30          Prob >= chibar2 = 0.0000
```

the fixed part of the regression model. This effect is −3.172244, which means that the score on the depression questionnaire is 3.17 points lower in the treatment group compared to the control group and adjusted for the differences in depression between the two groups at baseline. Around this treatment effect, the 95% CI ranges between −4.627396 and −1.717093, and the corresponding p-value is highly significant.

Output 11.2 Result of a linear IPD mixed model analysis to determine the effect of a treatment on depression adjusted for baseline differences and with a random intercept and a random slope for treatment on study level

```
Mixed-effects ML regression                Number of obs    =       574
Group variable: study                      Number of groups =         9

                                           Obs per group:
                                                        min =        47
                                                        avg =      63.8
                                                        max =        89

                                           Wald chi2(2)     =     78.79
Log likelihood = -2058.7203                Prob > chi2      =    0.0000

------------------------------------------------------------------------------
  depression |    Coef.   Std. Err.      z    P>|z|     [95% Conf. Interval]
-------------+----------------------------------------------------------------
   treatment | -3.080567   1.865654    -1.65   0.099    -6.737183    .576048
  depression0 |  .3945636   .0453465     8.70   0.000     .3056861   .4834411
       _cons |  7.629156   1.914596     3.98   0.000     3.876616    11.3817
------------------------------------------------------------------------------


------------------------------------------------------------------------------
  Random-effects Parameters  |   Estimate   Std. Err.     [95% Conf. Interval]
-----------------------------+------------------------------------------------
study: Unstructured          |
            var(treatm~n) |    26.5285    14.96737      8.7794    80.1605
              var(_cons) |   18.46956    9.960727     6.417991   53.1513
     cov(treatm~n,_cons) |  -18.40657   11.10617     -40.17426   3.361112
-----------------------------+------------------------------------------------
            var(Residual) |   72.05176    4.32171      64.06031   81.04015
------------------------------------------------------------------------------
LR test vs. linear model: chi2(3) = 58.70                Prob > chi2 = 0.0000
```

Because it is possible that the treatment effect is different for different studies, in the next step a random slope for treatment is added to the model. Output 11.2 shows the result of this analysis.

To evaluate whether a random slope for treatment was necessary, a likelihood ratio test can be performed to compare the model with only a random intercept with the model with both a random intercept and a random slope. Therefore, the difference between the two $-2\log$ likelihoods ($[-2 \times -2073.9191] - [-2 \times -2058.7023] = 30.43$) was calculated and evaluated on a Chi-square distribution with two degrees of freedom. The corresponding p-value is highly significant, so a random slope for treatment on study level is necessary. When a random slope significantly improves the model, it basically indicates that there is significant heterogeneity in the treatment effects between the studies. If the result of the analysis with only a random intercept (i.e. with only an adjustment for study) is compared with the result of the analysis with both a random intercept and a random slope for treatment, it can be seen that the estimated treatment effect is not much different between the two analyses. However, the standard error of the treatment effect is more than twice as high in the analysis with a random slope for treatment. This makes sense, because due to the heterogeneity in the estimated treatment effects between the studies, the combined treatment effect is estimated with less confidence (see also Chapter 3). Due to the increased standard error, the combined treatment effect, estimated with a mixed model analysis with a random intercept and a random slope for treatment on study level, was not statistically significant any more.

It is also possible that the adjustment for the baseline values is different for the different studies so, theoretically, a random slope for the baseline value of depression can also be added to the model. Output 11.3 shows the result of this analysis.

From Output 11.3 it can be seen that there is a problem in calculating the standard errors in the random part of the model. This problem is probably caused by the relatively low number of studies in this IPD meta-analysis. This potential problem has already been discussed in Chapter 2, and it was concluded that this does not have to be a big problem. So, ignoring the problems in estimating the standard errors, a likelihood ratio test can be performed to evaluate whether a random slope for the baseline value should be added to the model. The -2 log likelihood of the model without a random slope for the baseline value was $-2 \times -2058.7023 = 4117.4$, while the -2 log likelihood of the model with a random slope for the baseline value was $-2 \times -2053.5996 = 4107.2$. The difference between the two -2 log likelihoods equals 10.2 and must be evaluated on a Chi-square distribution with three degrees of freedom (i.e. the random slope for the baseline depression value, the covariance between random intercept and random slope for the baseline depression value, and the covariance between the random slope for treatment and the random slope for the baseline depression value), which is statistically significant.

It should be noted, however, that due to the problems in estimating the standard errors, in many situations the random slope for the baseline depression value will be removed from the final model. In that case the crude treatment effect of this one-stage IPD meta-analysis is derived from

Output 11.3 Result of a linear IPD mixed model analysis to determine the effect of a treatment on depression adjusted for baseline differences and with a random intercept, a random slope for treatment and a random slope for the baseline value on study level

```
Mixed-effects ML regression                    Number of obs      =         574
Group variable: study                          Number of groups   =           9

                                               Obs per group:
                                                          min =              47
                                                          avg =            63.8
                                                          max =              89

                                               Wald chi2(2)       =       42.96
Log likelihood = -2053.5996                    Prob > chi2        =      0.0000

------------------------------------------------------------------------------
  depression |     Coef.   Std. Err.      z    P>|z|    [95% Conf. Interval]
-------------+----------------------------------------------------------------
   treatment | -3.071712   1.863353    -1.65   0.099   -6.723816    .5803918
  depression0 |  .425176    .0651936     6.52   0.000    .297399     .552953
       _cons |  6.760002   1.589517     4.25   0.000    3.644606    9.875397
------------------------------------------------------------------------------


------------------------------------------------------------------------------
  Random-effects Parameters  |  Estimate   Std. Err.    [95% Conf. Interval]
-----------------------------+------------------------------------------------
study: Unstructured          |
               var(treatm~n) |   26.55229       .           .          .
               var(depres~0) |   .0180366       .           .          .
                 var(_cons)  |   7.612731       .           .          .
     cov(treatm~n,depres~0)  |  -.1806218       .           .          .
        cov(treatm~n,_cons)  |  -13.12751       .           .          .
        cov(depres~0,_cons)  |   -.048055       .           .          .
-----------------------------+------------------------------------------------
              var(Residual)  |   70.73147       .           .          .
------------------------------------------------------------------------------
LR test vs. linear model: chi2(6) = 68.94                Prob > chi2 = 0.0000
```

an analysis with a random intercept and a random slope for treatment on study level (see Output 11.2). This model will, therefore, be used as the crude model in the remaining part of this chapter. The overall treatment effect estimated with this model was −3.1, with a 95% CI ranging from −6.7 to 0.6 and with a corresponding p-value of 0.10.

One of the advantages of performing an IPD meta-analysis is that it is relatively easy to adjust the crude intervention effect for potential covariates and to investigate possible effect modification. This is done in the same way as has been described in the earlier chapters. For instance, an adjusted treatment effect in the example IPD meta-analysis can be estimated by adding the potential confounder(s) to the mixed model which was used for the estimation of the crude intervention effect. Output 11.4 shows the result of the IPD meta-analysis adjusted for age and gender.

Output 11.4 Result of a linear IPD mixed model analysis to determine the effect of a treatment on depression adjusted for baseline differences, age and gender and with a random intercept and random slope for treatment on study level

```
Mixed-effects ML regression                    Number of obs    =       574
Group variable: study                          Number of groups =         9

                                               Obs per group:
                                                            min =        47
                                                            avg =      63.8
                                                            max =        89

                                               Wald chi2(4)     =     79.37
Log likelihood = -2058.4647                    Prob > chi2      =    0.0000
```

depression	Coef.	Std. Err.	z	P>|z|	[95% Conf. Interval]	
treatment	-3.061399	1.866691	-1.64	0.101	-6.720046	.5972472
depression0	.3978557	.045661	8.71	0.000	.3083617	.4873497
age	-.0125963	.0289204	-0.44	0.663	-.0692793	.0440867
gender	-.5117872	.8665231	-0.59	0.555	-2.210141	1.186567
_cons	8.434721	2.313278	3.65	0.000	3.90078	12.96866

Random-effects Parameters	Estimate	Std. Err.	[95% Conf. Interval]	
study: Unstructured				
var(treatm~n)	26.55829	14.98732	8.787222	80.26913
var(_cons)	18.43266	9.949149	6.399506	53.09206
cov(treatm~n,_cons)	-18.38527	11.09895	-40.1388	3.368264
var(Residual)	71.98402	4.31769	64.00001	80.96405

```
LR test vs. linear model: chi2(3) = 58.50              Prob > chi2 = 0.0000
```

From Output 11.4 it can be seen that the adjustment for age and gender did not influence the regression coefficient for treatment. The adjusted treatment effect is more or less the same as the crude treatment effect. In the example dataset there are several other covariates available (i.e. marital status and education). However, both these covariates have some missing values, so when an analysis is performed with an adjustment for these two covariates, the sample on which the analysis is performed will be smaller than the sample used to estimate the crude treatment effect. The results of such an analysis should, therefore, be interpreted with caution. For illustration, Output 11.5 shows the result of an analysis in which an additional adjustment is performed for education and marital status.

From Output 11.5 it can be seen that in this adjusted analysis, only eight studies are involved, so this adjusted analysis cannot be compared with the crude analysis which was based on nine studies. From the result shown in Output 11.5 it can be seen that the treatment effect (-4.637198) is stronger than in the other analyses and, because of that, this adjusted treatment effect is also statistically significant ($p = 0.043$).

It should be noted that missing data can be a problem in IPD meta-analysis, because in general not all studies involved in the IPD meta-analysis measured the same variables. In the example used in this chapter, for instance, marital status was not measured in one of the nine

Output 11.5 Result of a linear IPD mixed model analysis to determine the effect of a treatment on depression adjusted for baseline differences, age, gender, education and marital status and with a random intercept and random slope for treatment on study level

```
Mixed-effects ML regression              Number of obs     =        467
Group variable: study                    Number of groups  =          8

                                         Obs per group:
                                                      min =         36
                                                      avg =       58.4
                                                      max =         89

                                         Wald chi2(8)      =      93.27
Log likelihood = -1662.1197              Prob > chi2       =     0.0000

-------------------------------------------------------------------------
 depression |    Coef.    Std. Err.      z    P>|z|    [95% Conf. Interval]
------------+------------------------------------------------------------
  treatment |  -4.637198   2.294144   -2.02   0.043   -9.133638  -.1407582
 depression0|   .4629625   .0509884    9.08   0.000    .363027    .562898
        age |  -.007079    .0325046   -0.22   0.828   -.0707868   .0566288
     gender |  -.7214172   .9460925   -0.76   0.446   -2.575725   1.13289
            |
  education |
   moderate |  -2.980571   1.761008   -1.69   0.091   -6.432083    .47094
       high |  -3.252102   1.800078   -1.81   0.071   -6.78019    .2759875
            |
maritalstatu|
     single |  -.5971075   .8865116   -0.67   0.501   -2.334638   1.140423
 divorced/~d|  -2.685182   1.245156   -2.16   0.031   -5.125643  -.2447208
            |
      _cons |   11.86068   3.082185    3.85   0.000    5.819705   17.90165
-------------------------------------------------------------------------


-------------------------------------------------------------------------
Random-effects Parameters    |   Estimate   Std. Err.    [95% Conf. Interval]
-----------------------------+-------------------------------------------
study: Unstructured          |
            var(treatm~n)    |   34.99061   21.64534    10.40866   117.6274
            var(_cons)       |   16.45732   10.39625    4.771411   56.76382
      cov(treatm~n,_cons)    |  -21.60817   14.21813   -49.47518    6.25885
-----------------------------+-------------------------------------------
            var(Residual)    |   68.35788   4.553638     59.991    77.89169
-------------------------------------------------------------------------
LR test vs. linear model: chi2(3) = 39.11              Prob > chi2 = 0.0000
```

studies. One of the solutions to get a full dataset is (multiple) imputation of missing values. How this imputation can best be performed goes beyond the scope of this book. For further information about multiple imputation for IPD meta-analysis see, for instance, Sterne et al. (2009), Donders et al. (2012), Jolani et al. (2015) and Audiger et al. (2017).

After estimating the adjusted treatment effect in this IPD meta-analysis, it can be investigated whether the estimated treatment effect is different for males and females, for instance, or for different ages, etc. To investigate this effect modification, the potential effect modifier and the interaction between treatment and the potential effect modifier must be added to the model. Output 11.6 shows the result of the analysis investigating possible effect modification by gender.

Output 11.6 Result of a linear IPD mixed model analysis to determine the effect of a treatment on depression adjusted for baseline differences and with an interaction between treatment and gender, and with a random intercept and random slope for treatment on study level

```
Mixed-effects ML regression                    Number of obs     =         574
Group variable: study                          Number of groups  =           9

                                               Obs per group:
                                                           min =          47
                                                           avg =        63.8
                                                           max =          89

                                               Wald chi2(4)      =       79.16
Log likelihood = -2058.5447                    Prob > chi2       =      0.0000

------------------------------------------------------------------------------
  depression |      Coef.   Std. Err.      z    P>|z|     [95% Conf. Interval]
-------------+----------------------------------------------------------------
 depression0 |   .3975711   .0456666     8.71   0.000     .3080662    .487076
   treatment |  -3.283694    2.27236    -1.45   0.148    -7.737438    1.17005
      gender |  -.6399593   1.22654     -0.52   0.602    -3.043934   1.764015
             |
c.treatment#|
    c.gender |    .293125   1.718014     0.17   0.865     -3.07412    3.66037
             |
       _cons |   8.024928   2.086078     3.85   0.000      3.93629   12.11357
------------------------------------------------------------------------------


------------------------------------------------------------------------------
  Random-effects Parameters  |   Estimate   Std. Err.     [95% Conf. Interval]
-----------------------------+------------------------------------------------
studyid: Unstructured        |
             var(treatm~n) |   26.51466   14.96279      8.77273    80.13777
               var(_cons) |   18.62951   10.03751      6.48003    53.55819
        cov(treatm~n,_cons) |  -18.48059   11.14489    -40.32417    3.362983
-----------------------------+------------------------------------------------
            var(Residual) |     71.998   4.318526      64.01244    80.97977
------------------------------------------------------------------------------
 LR test vs. linear model: chi2(3) = 58.93                Prob > chi2 = 0.0000
```

From Output 11.6 it can be seen that the interaction between treatment and gender is not statistically significant (p-value = 0.865), so there is no significant effect modification by gender, i.e. the combined treatment effect is not significantly different for males and females. The regression coefficient for treatment (3.283694) shown in Output 11.6 reflects the treatment effect for the group for which gender is coded 0 (i.e. males). The treatment effect for females can be calculated by adding the regression coefficient for treatment and the regression coefficient for the interaction between treatment and gender. The treatment effect for females is therefore −2.99 (−3.283694 + 0.293125). It should be noted that the interpretation of the results of an IPD meta-analysis to investigate whether the treatment effect is different for different groups is exactly the same as the interpretation of standard mixed model analyses with an interaction term, which is exactly the same as the interpretation of standard regression analysis with an interaction term (see also Chapter 7).

Output 11.7 shows the result of the analysis investigating possible effect modification by age.

From Output 11.7 it can be seen that there is no significant effect modification for age also. The p-value for the interaction term equals 0.965. The regression coefficient of treatment in Output 11.7 (−2.97669) now reflects the effect of the treatment for subjects with age equals zero, which is hardly informative because the age range in the example dataset goes from 18 to 79. The regression coefficient for the interaction term in Output 11.7 reflects the difference in treatment effect by one year difference in age. So, the treatment effect increases with increasing age, but again, this increase is far from significant.

11.3 **Comments**

There is a huge amount of literature dealing with IPD meta-analysis (Stewart and Parmar, 1993; Simmonds et al., 2005, 2015; Riley et al., 2010; Ahmed et al., 2011; Fischer et al., 2011; Cornell et al., 2014; Debray et al., 2015 and Burke et al., 2017) but, as has been mentioned before, a one-stage IPD meta-analysis is basically not much more than a mixed model analysis on individual data clustered within studies. The basic principles of mixed model analysis discussed in Chapter 2 also hold for a one-stage IPD meta-analysis. In the literature it is sometimes argued that a

Output 11.7 Result of a linear IPD mixed model analysis to determine the effect of a treatment on depression adjusted for baseline differences and with an interaction between treatment and age, and with a random intercept and random slope for treatment on study level

```
Mixed-effects ML regression                    Number of obs    =        574
Group variable: study                          Number of groups =          9

                                               Obs per group:
                                                          min =         47
                                                          avg =       63.8
                                                          max =         89

                                               Wald chi2(4)     =      79.00
Log likelihood = -2058.6379                    Prob > chi2      =     0.0000

------------------------------------------------------------------------------
  depression |      Coef.   Std. Err.      z    P>|z|     [95% Conf. Interval]
-------------+----------------------------------------------------------------
 depression0 |   .3947038   .0453493     8.70   0.000     .3058207    .4835869
   treatment |   -2.97669   3.002949    -0.99   0.322    -8.862362    2.908981
         age |  -.0103295   .0420435    -0.25   0.806    -.0927332    .0720742
             |
 c.treatment#|
      c.age  |  -.0025542   .0578721    -0.04   0.965    -.1159814     .110873
             |
       _cons |    8.04524   2.573913     3.13   0.002     3.000463    13.09002
------------------------------------------------------------------------------

------------------------------------------------------------------------------
  Random-effects Parameters  |   Estimate   Std. Err.     [95% Conf. Interval]
-----------------------------+------------------------------------------------
studyid: Unstructured        |
              var(treatm~n)  |   26.64461   15.04852      8.807687    80.60403
                var(_cons)   |   18.33987   9.913671      6.357357    52.90732
         cov(treatm~n,_cons) |  -18.37873   11.10783     -40.14967    3.392219
-----------------------------+------------------------------------------------
               var(Residual) |   72.03306   4.320709      64.04347    81.01938
------------------------------------------------------------------------------
LR test vs. linear model: chi2(3) = 57.83            Prob > chi2 = 0.0000
```

different estimation procedure must be used for IPD meta-analysis. Higgins et al. (2001), for instance, argue that a restricted maximum-likelihood estimation procedure must be used, especially when there are only a few studies involved in the meta-analysis and/or when the studies have relatively small sample sizes. In Chapter 2 the difference between maximum-likelihood estimation and restricted maximum-likelihood estimation was already mentioned, and it was concluded that the differences were rather small. To illustrate this difference within an IPD meta-analysis, Output 11.8 shows the results of the crude IPD meta-analysis (see Output 11.2) performed with a restricted maximum-likelihood estimation procedure.

Output 11.8 Result of a linear IPD mixed model analysis to determine the effect of a treatment on depression adjusted for baseline differences and with a random intercept and random slope for treatment on study level performed with restricted maximum likelihood

```
Mixed-effects REML regression              Number of obs     =       574
Group variable: study                      Number of groups  =         9

                                           Obs per group:
                                                        min =        47
                                                        avg =      63.8
                                                        max =        89

                                           Wald chi2(2)      =     77.99
Log restricted-likelihood = -2058.4982     Prob > chi2       =    0.0000

-------------------------------------------------------------------------
  depression |    Coef.    Std. Err.     z    P>|z|    [95% Conf. Interval]
-------------+-----------------------------------------------------------
   treatment | -3.074746   1.981842   -1.55   0.121   -6.959086   .8095934
  depression0|   .394192    .045435    8.68   0.000    .3051409    .483243
       _cons |  7.640536    1.99203    3.84   0.000     3.73623   11.54484
-------------------------------------------------------------------------


-------------------------------------------------------------------------
Random-effects Parameters    |   Estimate   Std. Err.    [95% Conf. Interval]
-----------------------------+-------------------------------------------
studyid: Unstructured        |
             var(treatm~n)   |  30.53685   17.88978     9.68622   96.27068
             var(_cons)      |  21.14082   11.90376    7.011904   63.73936
        cov(treatm~n,_cons)  | -21.08522   13.27908   -47.11173   4.941301
-----------------------------+-------------------------------------------
             var(Residual)   |  72.17769   4.332959    64.16583   81.18993
-------------------------------------------------------------------------
LR test vs. linear model: chi2(3) = 62.16              Prob > chi2 = 0.0000
```

If the result based on a restricted maximum-likelihood estimation procedure is compared to the result based on a maximum-likelihood estimation procedure (see Output 11.2), it can be seen that the estimations are only slightly different. The estimates of the combined treatment effect are almost equal, while the standard error estimated with restricted maximum likelihood is slightly higher than the standard error estimated with maximum likelihood.

In the literature it is also suggested that the estimated confidence interval of an IPD meta-analysis (both with maximum-likelihood and restricted maximum-likelihood estimation) is too small. They suggest to use the Kenward–Roger adjustment (Kenward and Roger, 1997), because it should better reflect the uncertainty in the effect estimate due to the heterogeneity between studies. Output 11.9 shows the result of the crude IPD meta-analysis with a Kenward–Roger adjustment.

Output 11.9 Result of a linear IPD mixed model analysis to determine the effect of a treatment on depression adjusted for baseline differences and with a random intercept and random slope for treatment on study level performed with restricted maximum likelihood and with a Kenward–Roger adjustment

```
Mixed-effects REML regression              Number of obs      =        574
Group variable: study                      Number of groups   =          9

                                           Obs per group:
                                                        min =         47
                                                        avg =       63.8
                                                        max =         89
DF method: Kenward-Roger                   DF:          min =       7.99
                                                        avg =     196.43
                                                        max =     563.19

                                           F(2,    20.29)     =      37.30
Log restricted-likelihood = -2058.4982     Prob > F           =     0.0000

------------------------------------------------------------------------------
  depression |     Coef.   Std. Err.      t    P>|t|     [95% Conf. Interval]
-------------+----------------------------------------------------------------
   treatment | -3.074746   1.982927    -1.55   0.160    -7.648602     1.49911
  depression0|   .394192    .0457258    8.62   0.000     .3043781    .4840059
       _cons |  7.640536   1.996325     3.83   0.001     3.448243    11.83283
------------------------------------------------------------------------------


------------------------------------------------------------------------------
  Random-effects Parameters  |   Estimate   Std. Err.     [95% Conf. Interval]
-----------------------------+------------------------------------------------
studyid: Unstructured        |
             var(treatm~n)   |   30.53685   17.88978      9.68622    96.27068
             var(_cons)      |   21.14082   11.90376      7.011904   63.73936
        cov(treatm~n,_cons)  |  -21.08522   13.27908    -47.11173    4.941301
-----------------------------+------------------------------------------------
             var(Residual)   |   72.17769    4.332959     64.16583   81.18993
------------------------------------------------------------------------------
LR test vs. linear model: chi2(3) = 62.16              Prob > chi2 = 0.0000
```

From Output 11.9 it can be seen that the confidence interval with the Kenward–Roger adjustment is wider than the confidence interval estimated in the regular way (known as the Dersimonian–Laird estimator). Therefore, the corresponding p-value is a bit higher.

It should be noted that, although the use of different estimation procedures make some sense, in practice most one-stage IPD meta-analysis are performed with a standard mixed model analysis. Also, this makes sense, because a one-stage IPD meta-analysis is nothing more than a regular mixed model analysis in which, for instance, subjects are clustered within neighbourhoods.

Sample-Size Calculations

12.1 Introduction

Before performing a study, some researchers believe that it is necessary to calculate the number of subjects that are needed in the study to make sure that a predefined effect will be statistically significant. It is necessary because sample-size calculations are a prerequisite for research grants and must be submitted to (medical) ethics committees. Furthermore, for experimental studies, sample-size calculations are part of the so-called CONSORT statement. This means that, without a sample-size calculation, a paper reporting the results of an experimental study will not be published in any of the major (medical) journals. It should be realised that the importance of sample-size calculations is highly questionable. First, sample-size calculations are based on many assumptions, which can easily be changed and in which case the number of subjects needed will be totally different. Second, sample-size calculations are based on testing theory (i.e. statistical testing and statistical significance). This is rather strange, because in epidemiological and medical research the importance of testing theory is becoming more and more questionable. Nevertheless, many people believe in the importance of sample-size calculations, and because standard sample-size calculations are not appropriate in mixed model studies, specific sample-size calculations must be used.

In general, to calculate the number of subjects or patients needed in a mixed model study, first a standard sample-size calculation must be performed and then a correction factor must be used. The problem, however, is that there are two potential correction factors available and that each leads to a (totally) different sample size.

12.2 Standard Sample-Size Calculations

Standard sample-size calculations are basically designed for experimental studies with one follow-up measurement. With this calculation the question answered is how many subjects are needed to get a certain predefined difference between the two groups statistically significant. Equation 12.1 shows the standard sample-size calculation for a continuous outcome variable.

$$N_1 = \frac{\left(Z_{(1-\alpha/2)} + Z_{(1-\beta)}\right)^2 \times \sigma^2 \times (r+1)}{v^2 \times r} \tag{12.1}$$

where N_1 = sample size for the intervention group, α = significance level, $Z_{(1-\alpha/2)}$ = $(1 - \alpha/2)$ percentile point of the standard normal distribution, $(1 - \beta)$ = power, $Z_{(1-\beta)}$ = $(1 - \beta)$ percentile point of the standard normal distribution, σ = standard deviation of the outcome variable, r = ratio of the number of subjects in the groups compared, i.e. N_0/N_1, N_0 = sample size for the control group and v = difference in mean value of the outcome variable between the groups.

A comparable equation can be used for dichotomous outcome variables (Eq. 12.2).

$$N_1 = \frac{\left(Z_{(1-\alpha/2)} + Z_{(1-\beta)}\right)^2 \times \bar{p}(1 - \bar{p}) \times (r+1)}{\left(p_1 - p_0\right)^2 \times r} \tag{12.2a}$$

$$\bar{p} = \frac{p_1 + (r \times p_0)}{1 + r} \tag{12.2b}$$

where N_1 = sample size for the intervention group, α = significance level, $Z_{(1-\alpha/2)}$ = $(1 - \alpha/2)$ percentile point of the standard normal distribution, $(1 - \beta)$ = power; $Z_{(1-\beta)}$ = $(1 - \beta)$ percentile point of the standard normal distribution; $\bar{p}$ = average of p_0 and p_1, r = ratio of the number of subjects in the groups compared, i.e. N_0/N_1, N_0 = sample size for the control group, p_1 = proportion of cases in the intervention group and p_0 = proportion of cases in the control group.

12.3 Sample-Size Calculations for Mixed Model Studies

As has been mentioned before, there are two different correction factors that can be used to calculate the required sample size in mixed model studies. Equation 12.3 shows the first correction factor, which is known as the conservative correction factor:

$$m \times n = N \times [1 + (n - 1)\rho] \qquad (12.3)$$

where N = number of subjects according to the standard sample-size calculation, m = number of clusters (number of neighbourhoods, number of GPs, number of schools, etc.), n = number of observations for each cluster and ρ = intraclass correlation coefficient.

It is also possible to calculate the relative effectiveness of a certain sample size when that sample size is applied in a mixed model study (Eq. 12.4).

$$N_{\text{effective}} = \frac{N}{[1 + (n - 1)\rho]} \qquad (12.4)$$

where $N_{\text{effective}}$ = effective sample size by a given standard sample size (based on m times n observations).

Equation 12.5 shows the second correction factor, which is known as the liberal correction factor, that can be used to calculate the required sample size for a mixed model study. Equation 12.6 shows the corresponding equation to calculate the effective sample size.

$$m = \frac{N}{1 + (n - 1)(1 - \rho)} \qquad (12.5)$$

$$N_{\text{effective}} = m \times [1 + (n - 1)(1 - \rho)] \qquad (12.6)$$

12.4 Example

Suppose that a sample-size calculation is performed for an intervention study in which the patients are clustered within GPs, and that with a standard sample-size calculation it is calculated that 100 patients are needed in each group. Suppose further that for each GP 10 patients are included, and that the intraclass correlation coefficient (ICC) for patients within GPs equals 0.2. When those numbers are added to Eq. 12.3 (i.e. the conservative correction factor), it can be calculated that 28 GPs are needed; so instead of 100 patients, in a mixed model situation with a relatively small ICC of 0.2, 280 patients are needed. However, if those numbers are added to Eq. 12.5 (i.e. the liberal correction factor), it can be calculated that 12.2 GPs are needed, which means a sample-size of 122 patients instead of 100.

When the effective sample sizes are calculated in this situation (i.e. 100 patients, 10 GPs and an ICC of 0.2), the effective sample size calculated with the conservative correction factor (Eq. 12.4) equals 35.7. Calculated with the liberal correction factor (Eq. 12.6), on the other hand, the effective sample size equals 82.

12.5 Which Sample-Size Calculation Should Be Used?

The two correction factors that can be used to calculate the sample size for a mixed model study lead to totally different results, and the questions 'Which one is better?' and 'Which one should be used?' arise. The way in which the two correction factors differ from each other can best be illustrated by a small example. Suppose the ICC in a certain mixed model study is 0.20. For the conservative procedure this means that the first subject in a certain cluster provides 100% new information, and the second subject in that cluster provides 80% new information. The third subject in that cluster also provides 80% new information; however, not of the original 100%, but of the remaining 80%, which implies that the third subject only provides 64% new information. In the same way, the fourth subject in that cluster only provides 51% new information (i.e. 80% of 64%), and so on. This implies that when the number of subjects increases for a certain cluster, almost no new information is obtained.

As for the conservative correction factor, the first subject for the liberal correction factor provides 100% new information and the second subject also provides 80% new information. However, the difference between the two correction factors is that for the liberal correction factor all other subjects in the cluster also provide 80% new information. So, the third subject provides 80% new information, the fourth subject provides 80% new information, and so on.

To answer the question concerning which of the two correction factors should be applied, the example in Chapter 3 will be used. The example used in that chapter showed that in a naive analysis with 200 patients an intervention effect of 0.289 was found, with a corresponding standard error of 0.121 (see Output 3.2). When a random intercept and a random slope for the intervention variable were added to the model, the magnitude of the intervention effect remained the same (0.289), but the standard error increased to 0.175 (see Output 3.4). The ICC in this example was approximately 0.43. When the two sample-size correction factors are applied to this example, according to the conservative correction factor 974 patients are needed to obtain the same efficiency/power as the naive analysis with 200 patients, while with the liberal correction factor only 380 patients are needed. Looking at the two standard errors of the naive analysis and the mixed model analysis, it can be seen that the standard error in the analysis with a random intercept and a random slope is 1.45 times higher than the standard error in the naive analysis. If this is related to the increase in sample size, it means that $(1.45)^2 = 2.1$ times more patients are needed to obtain the same efficiency/power. In other words, 420 patients are needed in the analysis with a random intercept and random slope to obtain the same efficiency/power as in the naive analysis. When these 420 patients are compared to the sample sizes calculated with the two correction factors, it can be seen that the conservative correction factor leads to a huge overestimation, while the liberal correction factor leads to a slight underestimation.

In the above example the randomisation was performed on patient level, but when the randomisation is performed on GP level (i.e. a cluster randomisation), the situation is different. Table 3.1 summarised the results of the analysis on the example dataset in which cluster randomisation was used. Output 12.1 and Output 12.2 show the results of these analyses in greater detail. Output 12.1 shows the result of a naive analysis to estimate the intervention effect in this situation, while Output 12.2 shows the result of the corresponding mixed model analysis. Note that, because the randomisation was performed on GP level, only a random intercept could be added to the model.

From Output 12.2 it can be calculated that the ICC in this example is approximately 0.23 $(0.17/(0.17 + 0.56) = 0.2329)$. When this ICC is added to the sample-size equations, with the conservative correction factor

Output 12.1 Result of a naive analysis performed on a (balanced) dataset regarding the relationship between the intervention and health, when the randomisation was performed on GP level

```
Mixed-effects ML regression                  Number of obs    =        200

                                             Wald chi2(1)     =       4.58
Log likelihood = -252.42434                  Prob > chi2      =     0.0324

------------------------------------------------------------------------------
      health |     Coef.   Std. Err.      z    P>|z|     [95% Conf. Interval]
-------------+----------------------------------------------------------------
intervention |     .2586   .1208955     2.14   0.032     .0216491    .4955509
       _cons |    6.5166   .0854861    76.23   0.000      6.34905    6.68415
------------------------------------------------------------------------------


------------------------------------------------------------------------------
  Random-effects Parameters |   Estimate   Std. Err.    [95% Conf. Interval]
-----------------------------+------------------------------------------------
                var(Residual)|  .7307867   .0730787    .6007178    .8890185
------------------------------------------------------------------------------
```

Output 12.2 Result of a mixed model analysis on a (balanced) dataset regarding the relationship between the intervention and health, with a random intercept, when the randomisation was performed on GP level

```
Mixed-effects ML regression                  Number of obs    =        200
Group variable: gp                           Number of groups =         20

                                             Obs per group:
                                                          min =         10
                                                          avg =       10.0
                                                          max =         10

                                             Wald chi2(1)     =       1.47
Log likelihood = -239.77215                  Prob > chi2      =     0.2248

------------------------------------------------------------------------------
      health |     Coef.   Std. Err.      z    P>|z|     [95% Conf. Interval]
-------------+----------------------------------------------------------------
intervention |     .2586   .2130435     1.21   0.225    -.1589576    .6761576
       _cons |    6.5166   .1506445    43.26   0.000     6.221342    6.811858
------------------------------------------------------------------------------


------------------------------------------------------------------------------
  Random-effects Parameters |   Estimate   Std. Err.    [95% Conf. Interval]
-----------------------------+------------------------------------------------
gp: Identity                 |
                var(_cons)   |  .1709544   .0720062    .0748778    .3903081
-----------------------------+------------------------------------------------
                var(Residual)|  .5598324   .0590115    .4553376    .6883076
------------------------------------------------------------------------------
LR test vs. linear model: chibar2(01) = 25.30        Prob >= chibar2 = 0.0000
```

614 patients are needed, while with the liberal correction factor only 252 patients are needed. From both outputs it can further be seen that the intervention effect is equal (0.259), but compared to the naive analysis the standard error of the intervention effect increased in the mixed model analysis from 0.121 to 0.213, which is 1.76 times higher. If this increase in the standard error is related to the increase in sample size, it means that $(1.76)^2 = 3.1$ times more patients are needed to obtain the same efficiency/power in the mixed model analysis as in the naive analysis. In other words, when the randomisation is performed on GP level, 620 patients are needed in the analysis with a random intercept to obtain the same efficiency/power as in the naive analysis. So, in this situation the conservative correction factor is almost perfect, while the liberal correction factor leads to a huge underestimation of the required sample size.

12.6 Comments

It should be noted that with the sample-size calculations the number of clusters (noted as m) can be estimated. In most studies, however, the number of clusters (e.g. the number of GPs) that can be included in a study is not very flexible, and the question that must be answered is: how many patients should be included for each GP? When using the conservative correction factor there is a problem, because the sampling of more patients within a GP is of little use. At a certain point, depending on the magnitude of the ICC, a new patient provides almost no new information. With the liberal correction factor, however, sampling more patients for each GP is a potential way of increasing the efficiency/power of a mixed model study.

In fact, when designing a mixed model study, the most appropriate combination of the number of clusters and the number of subjects within a cluster must be calculated (Snijders and Bosker, 1993; Lee and Durbin, 1994; Liu and Liang, 1997; Plewis and Hurry, 1998; Hedeker et al, 1999; Moerbeek et al, 2000, 2003b; Jung et al., 2001). In general, the more clusters that are included in a study, the better. When the number of clusters is high in relation to the number of subjects within a cluster, there is less influence of the correlation between the observations within one cluster. However, it has already been mentioned that, theoretically, the most appropriate combination can be calculated, but in most practical situations this will be very difficult to achieve.

In real-life practice, researchers often use a different sample-size adjustment to take into account the correlation of the observations within clusters. Suppose that the calculated sample size is 100 and that the assumed ICC will be 0.10. The corrected sample size will then be 10% more, which in this case is 110. When the ICC is assumed to be 0.20, the corrected sample size will be 20% more, which will lead to a corrected sample size of 120. From the earlier reported results of the different sample-size calculations, it can be seen that this very simple correction is comparable to the liberal sample-size correction factor and therefore an underestimation of the sample size that is needed to get a certain predefined difference statistically significant.

It should be realised that for sample-size calculations certain assumptions are necessary with regard to the expected difference between the groups, the standard deviation of the outcome variable of interest, the power of the study and the ICC. Furthermore, it has already been mentioned that sample-size calculations are based on testing theory (i.e. statistical testing and statistical significance), the importance of which is highly questionable. Because of these issues, the importance of sample-size calculations is rather limited, and therefore sample-size calculations should be used with great caution.

13

Some Loose Ends . . .

In this last chapter some loose ends will be tightened. First, the *xt* procedure in STATA will be discussed. With the *xt* procedure, mixed model analysis with only a random intercept can be performed for many different outcome variables. The *xt* procedure can also be used to analyse hybrid models (see Section 13.2). Finally, the performance of different software programs will be discussed.

13.1 The *xt* Procedures in STATA

In the foregoing chapters several possibilities for performing mixed model analyses for different outcome variables have been discussed. Within STATA there are *xt* procedures available, with which it is possible to perform mixed model analyses with only a random intercept. The simplest *xt* procedure is *xtreg*, which is basically the same as the *mixed* procedure with only a random intercept used in the foregoing chapters. To illustrate the use of the *xt* procedure, Output 13.1 and Output 13.2 show the results of analyses of the relationship between physical activity and health (the example used in Chapter 2) with a random intercept on neighbourhood level performed with the *xtreg* procedure (Output 13.1) and with the *mixed* procedure (Output 13.2)

From Output 13.1 and Output 13.2 it can be seen that both procedures lead to exactly the same results in both the fixed part of the model and the random part of the model. It should be noted that with the *xtreg* procedure (Output 13.1) instead of the random intercept and residual variances, the standard deviations are given. Furthermore, the output of the *xtreg*

Output 13.1 Result of an analysis of the relationship between physical activity and health, with a random intercept on neighbourhood level performed with the *xtreg* procedure

```
Random-effects ML regression                Number of obs     =        684
Group variable: neighbourhood               Number of groups  =         48

Random effects u_i ~ Gaussian               Obs per group:
                                                          min =          4
                                                          avg =       14.3
                                                          max =         49

                                            LR chi2(1)        =     206.82
Log likelihood  = -2153.4088                Prob > chi2       =     0.0000

-------------------------------------------------------------------------------
      health |      Coef.   Std. Err.      z    P>|z|     [95% Conf. Interval]
-------------+-----------------------------------------------------------------
    activity |   .5896818   .0379472    15.54   0.000     .5153068    .6640569
       _cons |   .7898843   1.941144     0.41   0.684    -3.014688    4.594456
-------------+-----------------------------------------------------------------
     /sigma_u |  2.004674   .3391293                      1.438953    2.792807
     /sigma_e |  5.438711   .1527519                      5.147414    5.746493
         rho |   .1196107   .0367721                      .0620184    .207301
-------------------------------------------------------------------------------
LR test of sigma_u=0: chibar2(01) = 30.96             Prob >= chibar2 = 0.000
```

Output 13.2 Result of a mixed model analysis of the relationship between physical activity and health, with a random intercept on neighbourhood level performed with the *mixed* procedure

```
Mixed-effects ML regression                 Number of obs     =        684
Group variable: neighbourhood               Number of groups  =         48

                                            Obs per group:
                                                          min =          4
                                                          avg =       14.3
                                                          max =         49

                                            Wald chi2(1)      =     241.50
Log likelihood = -2153.4088                 Prob > chi2       =     0.0000

-------------------------------------------------------------------------------
      health |      Coef.   Std. Err.      z    P>|z|     [95% Conf. Interval]
-------------+-----------------------------------------------------------------
    activity |   .5896818    .037945    15.54   0.000      .515311    .6640527
       _cons |   .7898844   1.941018     0.41   0.684     -3.01444    4.594209
-------------------------------------------------------------------------------

-------------------------------------------------------------------------------
  Random-effects Parameters   |   Estimate   Std. Err.    [95% Conf. Interval]
-----------------------------+-------------------------------------------------
neighbourh~d: Identity       |
                var(_cons)   |   4.018727   1.359694      2.070587    7.799802
-----------------------------+-------------------------------------------------
               var(Residual) |  29.57958   1.661547      26.49587    33.02218
-------------------------------------------------------------------------------
LR test vs. linear model: chibar2(01) = 30.96        Prob >= chibar2 = 0.0000
```

procedure directly provides an estimation of the ICC (0.1196107). Besides that, in the *mixed* procedure, the Wald statistic is used to obtain the overall *p*-value, while in the *xtreg* procedure the likelihood ratio test is used. It is known that both tests lead to slightly different results. However, this is not really important, because the overall *p*-value for the whole model is not used much in practice.

Comparable to a linear mixed model analysis, it is also possible to use the *xtlogit* procedure to perform a logistic mixed model analysis. Output 13.3 and Output 13.4 show the results of analyses of the relationship between physical activity and the dichotomous health indicator (the example used in Chapter 4), with a random intercept on neighbourhood level performed with the *xtlogit* procedure (Output 13.3) and the *melogit* procedure (Output 13.4).

From Output 13.3 and Output 13.4 it can be seen that both procedures lead to exactly the same results. Again, the *xtlogit* procedure provides standard deviations instead of variances for the random part of the model and the *xtlogit* procedure provides a /*lnsig2u*, which is the natural log of the

Output 13.3 Results of a mixed model analysis of the relationship between physical activity and the dichotomous health indicator with a random intercept on neighbourhood level performed with the *xtlogit* procedure

```
Random-effects logistic regression              Number of obs     =        684
Group variable: neighbourhood                   Number of groups  =         48

Random effects u_i ~ Gaussian                   Obs per group:
                                                             min =          4
                                                             avg =       14.3
                                                             max =         49

Integration method: mvaghermite                 Integration pts.  =         12

                                                Wald chi2(1)      =      83.43
Log likelihood  = -408.96782                    Prob > chi2       =     0.0000

------------------------------------------------------------------------------
health_dich |      Coef.   Std. Err.      z    P>|z|     [95% Conf. Interval]
------------+-----------------------------------------------------------------
   activity |   .1685528   .0184534     9.13   0.000     .1323848    .2047207
      _cons |  -8.243315   .9319367    -8.85   0.000    -10.06988   -6.416753
------------+-----------------------------------------------------------------
   /lnsig2u |  -.7201464   .4462502                     -1.594781    .1544878
------------+-----------------------------------------------------------------
    sigma_u |   .6976252   .1556577                      .4505031   1.080306
        rho |   .1288692   .0500969                      .0581058    .261853
------------------------------------------------------------------------------
LR test of rho=0: chibar2(01) = 16.60                   Prob >= chibar2 = 0.000
```

Output 13.4 Results of a mixed model analysis of the relationship between physical activity and the dichotomous health indicator with a random intercept on neighbourhood level performed with the *melogit* procedure

```
Mixed-effects logistic regression          Number of obs    =       684
Group variable:  neighbourhood             Number of groups =        48

                                           Obs per group:
                                                        min =         4
                                                        avg =      14.3
                                                        max =        49

Integration method: mvaghermite            Integration pts. =         7

                                           Wald chi2(1)     =     83.43
Log likelihood = -408.96783                Prob > chi2      =    0.0000
-------------+------------------------------------------------------------
 health_dich |    Coef.   Std. Err.     z    P>|z|    [95% Conf. Interval]
-------------+------------------------------------------------------------
    activity |  .1685528   .0184534    9.13   0.000    .1323849    .2047207
       _cons | -8.243316   .9319357   -8.85   0.000   -10.06988   -6.416756
-------------+------------------------------------------------------------
neighbourhood |
   var(_cons)|  .4866812   .2171715                    .2029613    1.167013
-------------+------------------------------------------------------------
LR test vs. logistic model: chibar2(01) = 16.60       Prob >= chibar2 = 0.0000
```

Table 13.1 Examples of *xt* procedures that can be used for mixed model analysis with a random intercept for different outcome variables

xtpoisson	Poisson regression analysis (see Chapter 5)
xtnegbin	Negative binomial regression analysis (see Chapter 5)
xtgee	Generalised estimating equations (see Chapters 4 and 9)
xttobit	Tobit regression analysis, i.e. regression analysis for outcome variables with floor and/or ceiling effects
xtstreg	Parametric survival analysis (see Chapter 5)

random intercept variance, which is not really informative. Surprisingly, the *xtlogit* procedure also provides an ICC (0.1288692). This ICC is comparable to the one calculated in Chapter 4 with Eq. 4.1 (see Section 4.3). Furthermore, it can be seen that for the logistic mixed model analysis, both procedures use the Wald statistic to obtain the overall *p*-value for the model.

As has been mentioned before, there are many other outcome variables that can be analysed with an *xt* procedure. Table 13.1 shows a few examples.

For further details about the *xtreg* procedure one is referred to the STATA software manual.

13.2 Hybrid Models Revisited

When a longitudinal data analysis is performed, the effect estimate combines the between-subject part and the within-subject part of the relationship into one coefficient (see Section 9.2). In Section 9.3 hybrid models were introduced as a possible way to disentangle the between-subject part and the within-subject part of the relationship. It was mentioned that the between-subject part is basically nothing more than the relationship between the mean value of the particular independent variable for each subject and the time-dependent outcome variable. To obtain the within-subject part of the relationship, the independent variable has to be centred around the mean of the particular subject. The difference between the observations at each time point and the subjects' mean value is known as the deviation score and reflects the within-subject part of the longitudinal relationship. In Section 9.4 both variables were calculated and analysed with a mixed model analysis. In STATA it is, however, also possible to obtain the within-subject part and the between-subject part of the longitudinal relationship directly from the *xtreg* procedure. When *fe* is added to the *xtreg* procedure, the within-subject part of the relationship is estimated, while with *be* the *xtreg* procedure provides the between-subject part of the relationship. It should be noted that *fe* stands for fixed effect. This is rather confusing, because in mixed model analysis a distinction is made between the fixed part of the regression model and the random part of the regression model. The fixed part of the regression model is the part in which the regression coefficients are given, which is different from the within-subject part of the relationship reflected by the *fe* option.

To illustrate the use of these procedures, the example used in Section 9.4 (which the longitudinal relationship between lifestyle and health was analysed) will be used. Output 13.5 shows the results of the mixed (hybrid) model analysis to analyse this relationship.

From Output 13.5 it can be seen that the regression coefficient reflecting the between-subject part of the relationship equals 0.1593343 and the regression coefficient reflecting the within-subject part of the relationship equals 0.01624. As has been mentioned before, these two effects can also be obtained with the *xtreg* procedure. Output 13.6 and Output 13.7 show the results of these analyses.

Output 13.5 Result of a linear mixed (hybrid) model analysis of the longitudinal relationship between lifestyle and health with a random intercept on subject level

```
Mixed-effects ML regression                 Number of obs     =        588
Group variable: subject                     Number of groups  =        147

                                            Obs per group:
                                                          min =          4
                                                          avg =        4.0
                                                          max =          4

                                            Wald chi2(2)      =      19.07
Log likelihood = -401.41979                 Prob > chi2       =     0.0001

------------------------------------------------------------------------------
      health |     Coef.   Std. Err.      z    P>|z|    [95% Conf. Interval]
-------------+----------------------------------------------------------------
mean_lifest~e | .1593343   .0367842     4.33   0.000    .0872385    .2314301
dev_lifestyle |   .01624   .029167      0.56   0.578   -.0409262    .0734062
        _cons | 3.743517   .1370168    27.32   0.000    3.474969    4.012064
------------------------------------------------------------------------------


------------------------------------------------------------------------------
  Random-effects Parameters  |   Estimate   Std. Err.    [95% Conf. Interval]
-----------------------------+------------------------------------------------
subject: Identity            |
                var(_cons)   |   .3077503   .0396512      .2390715    .3961587
-----------------------------+------------------------------------------------
               var(Residual) |   .1267816   .0085379      .1111049    .1446702
------------------------------------------------------------------------------
LR test vs. linear model: chibar2(01) = 375.74      Prob >= chibar2 = 0.0000
```

Output 13.6 Result of a linear mixed model analysis of the between-subject relationship between lifestyle and health with a random intercept on subject level

```
Between regression (regression on group means)  Number of obs     =      588
Group variable: subject                         Number of groups  =      147

R-sq:                                           Obs per group:
    within  = 0.0007                                          min =        4
    between = 0.1132                                          avg =      4.0
    overall = 0.0813                                          max =        4

                                                F(1,145)          =    18.51
sd(u_i + avg(e_i.))=   .586624                  Prob > F          =   0.0000

------------------------------------------------------------------------------
      health |     Coef.   Std. Err.      t    P>|t|    [95% Conf. Interval]
-------------+----------------------------------------------------------------
   lifestyle | .1593343   .0370371     4.30   0.000    .0861321    .2325366
       _cons | 3.743517   .1379585    27.14   0.000    3.470847    4.016186
------------------------------------------------------------------------------
```

Output 13.7 Results of a linear mixed model analysis of the within-subject relationship between lifestyle and health with a random intercept on subject level

```
Fixed-effects (within) regression          Number of obs   =       588
Group variable: subject                    Number of groups =      147

R-sq:                                      Obs per group:
    within  = 0.0007                                    min =         4
    between = 0.1132                                    avg =       4.0
    overall = 0.0813                                    max =         4

                                           F(1,440)        =      0.31
corr(u_i, Xb)  = 0.2851                    Prob > F        =    0.5784

------------------------------------------------------------------------
      health |    Coef.   Std. Err.      t    P>|t|   [95% Conf. Interval]
-------------+----------------------------------------------------------
   lifestyle |   .01624   .0292001     0.56   0.578   -.041149    .073629
       _cons |  4.24267   .1029135    41.23   0.000   4.040407   4.444933
-------------+----------------------------------------------------------
     sigma_u |  .6139659
     sigma_e |  .35646846
         rho |  .74788941   (fraction of variance due to u_i)
------------------------------------------------------------------------
F test that all u_i=0: F(146, 440) = 10.90            Prob > F = 0.0000
```

From Output 13.6 and Output 13.7 it can be seen that the two regression coefficients are exactly the same as the regression coefficients obtained from the hybrid mixed model analysis shown in Output 13.5. The standard errors, however, are slightly different between the two procedures as are the random intercept variance and the residual variance. It can further be seen that the *xtreg* procedure provides some additional information which is not provided by the *mixed* procedure: the explained variances of the within-subject part and the between-subject part of the relationship, an estimation of the residual standard deviation (0.586624) and the correlation between the regression coefficient for the within-subject part of the relationship and the corresponding random effect (0.2851). However, this additional information is not very useful.

In this section the *xtreg* procedure is used to disentangle the within-subject part and the between-subject part of a longitudinal relationship. Although less frequently used, the same procedure can also be used for cross-sectional analysis in which the outcome variable of interest is, for instance, clustered within neighbourhoods. To illustrate this, the example of Chapter 2 will be used, in which the relationship between physical activity and health was investigated. In this example the outcome variable health was clustered within 48 neighbourhoods. Output 13.8 shows the result of the

Output 13.8 Result of a linear mixed model analysis of the relationship between physical activity and health, with a random intercept on neighbourhood level

```
Mixed-effects ML regression              Number of obs     =         684
Group variable: neighbourhood            Number of groups  =          48

                                         Obs per group:
                                                       min =           4
                                                       avg =        14.3
                                                       max =          49

                                         Wald chi2(1)      =      241.50
Log likelihood = -2153.4088              Prob > chi2       =      0.0000

-----------------------------------------------------------------------------
      health |     Coef.    Std. Err.      z     P>|z|    [95% Conf. Interval]
-------------+---------------------------------------------------------------
    activity |   .5896818    .037945    15.54    0.000     .515311     .6640527
       _cons |   .7898844   1.941018     0.41    0.684    -3:01444    4.594209
-----------------------------------------------------------------------------


-----------------------------------------------------------------------------
  Random-effects Parameters   |   Estimate   Std. Err.    [95% Conf. Interval]
------------------------------+----------------------------------------------
neighbourh~d: Identity        |
                 var(_cons)   |   4.018727   1.359694     2.070587    7.799802
------------------------------+----------------------------------------------
               var(Residual)  |   29.57958   1.661547    26.49587    33.02218
-----------------------------------------------------------------------------
LR test vs. linear model: chibar2(01) = 30.96        Prob >= chibar2 = 0.0000
```

Output 13.9 Result of a linear mixed model analysis of the between-neighbourhood relationship between physical activity and health with a random intercept on neighbourhood level

```
Between regression (regression on group means)  Number of obs     =       684
Group variable: neighbourh~d                    Number of groups  =        48

R-sq:                                           Obs per group:
    within  = 0.2611                                          min =         4
    between = 0.2737                                          avg =      14.3
    overall = 0.2607                                          max =        49

                                                F(1,46)           =     17.33
sd(u_i + avg(e_i.))=  2.731655                  Prob > F          =    0.0001

-----------------------------------------------------------------------------
      health |     Coef.    Std. Err.      t     P>|t|    [95% Conf. Interval]
-------------+---------------------------------------------------------------
    activity |   .6468726   .1553813     4.16    0.000     .3341063    .9596389
       _cons |  -2.069951   7.822985    -0.26    0.793    -17.8168    13.6769
-----------------------------------------------------------------------------
```

mixed model analysis to analyse the relationship between physical activity and health with a random intercept on neighbourhood level.

Output 13.9 and Output 13.10 show the result of the linear mixed model analysis to obtain the between-neighbourhood part of the relationship

Output 13.10 Results of a linear mixed model analysis of the within-neighbourhood relationship between physical activity and health with a random intercept on neighbourhood level

```
Fixed-effects (within) regression          Number of obs      =        684
Group variable: neighbourh~d               Number of groups   =         48

R-sq:                                      Obs per group:
    within  = 0.2611                                     min =          4
    between = 0.2737                                     avg =       14.3
    overall = 0.2607                                     max =         49

                                           F(1,635)           =     224.33
corr(u_i, Xb)  = 0.0156                     Prob > F           =     0.0000

-------------------------------------------------------------------------------
    health |      Coef.   Std. Err.      t    P>|t|     [95% Conf. Interval]
-----------+-------------------------------------------------------------------
  activity |   .5868455   .0391816    14.98   0.000     .5099044    .6637866
     _cons |   .9022762   1.976451     0.46   0.648    -2.978895    4.783447
-----------+-------------------------------------------------------------------
   sigma_u |  2.7068189
   sigma_e |  5.4356245
       rho |   .19870615   (fraction of variance due to u_i)
-------------------------------------------------------------------------------
F test that all u_i=0: F(47, 635) = 2.86               Prob > F = 0.0000
```

(Output 13.9) and the result of the linear mixed model analysis to obtain the within-neighbourhood part of the relationship.

From Output 13.9 and Output 13.10 it can be seen that the between-neighbourhood relationship between physical activity and health is slightly higher than the within-neighbourhood relationship. It should be noted that the use of hybrid models in cross-sectional studies is not widely used in real-life practice.

13.3 Bayesian Mixed Model Analysis

13.3.1 Introduction

The last few years have seen a growing interest in using Bayesian methods to analyse mixed model data. Basically, there are two main differences between the standard mixed model analysis and the Bayesian mixed model analysis. First, the parameters of interest are not fixed but are random and estimated from a posterior distribution. Second, the posterior distribution of the parameters of interest can be influenced by certain information derived from other studies or from the literature. The latter is known as prior information. The general idea of Bayesian mixed model analysis is that the prior information is combined with the observed data to obtain the posterior distribution of the parameters of interest. Based on the posterior distribution point, estimates such as the average, the median and credible intervals can be derived. The credible interval is the Bayesian counterpart of the confidence interval. To illustrate the differences between the standard mixed model analysis and the Bayesian mixed model analysis, we reanalysed the example data of Chapter 2 with both methods. In the example the relationship between physical activity and health was investigated. Because the 648 subjects were living in 48 neighbourhoods, a random intercept on neighbourhood level was added to the model. Output 13.11 and Output 13.12 show the results of the analyses.

The output of the Bayesian mixed model analysis is a bit more extensive compared to the output of the standard mixed model analysis. The first part of the Bayesian output contains information of the prior distributions used in the analysis, while the second part of the Bayesian output contains

Output 13.11 Results of a linear mixed model analysis of the relationship between physical activity and health, with a random intercept on neighbourhood level

```
Mixed-effects ML regression                      Number of obs     =        684
Group variable: neighbourhood                    Number of groups  =         48

                                                 Obs per group:
                                                              min =          4
                                                              avg =       14.3
                                                              max =         49

                                                 Wald chi2(1)      =     241.50
Log likelihood = -2153.4088                      Prob > chi2       =     0.0000

------------------------------------------------------------------------------
      health |      Coef.   Std. Err.      z    P>|z|     [95% Conf. Interval]
-------------+----------------------------------------------------------------
    activity |   .5896818    .037945    15.54   0.000     .515311    .6640527
       _cons |   .7898844   1.941018     0.41   0.684    -3.01444   4.594209
------------------------------------------------------------------------------

------------------------------------------------------------------------------
  Random-effects Parameters  |   Estimate   Std. Err.     [95% Conf. Interval]
-----------------------------+------------------------------------------------
neighbourh~d: Identity       |
                 var(_cons)  |   4.018727   1.359694     2.070587    7.799802
-----------------------------+------------------------------------------------
               var(Residual) |   29.57958   1.661547     26.49587    33.02218
------------------------------------------------------------------------------
LR test vs. linear model: chibar2(01) = 30.96          Prob >= chibar2 = 0.0000
```

Output 13.12 Results of a Bayesian linear mixed model analysis of the relationship between physical activity and health, with a random intercept on neighbourhood level

```
Multilevel structure
-------------------------------------------------------------------------------
neighbourhood
     {U0}: random intercepts
-------------------------------------------------------------------------------

Model summary
-------------------------------------------------------------------------------
Likelihood:
  health ~ normal(xb_health,{e.health:sigma2})

Priors:
  {health:activity _cons} ~ normal(0,10000)                                  (1)
                  {U0} ~ normal(0,{U0:sigma2})                              (1)
      {e.health:sigma2} ~ igamma(.01,.01)

Hyperprior:
  {U0:sigma2} ~ igamma(.01,.01)
-------------------------------------------------------------------------------
(1) Parameters are elements of the linear form xb_health.

Bayesian multilevel regression              MCMC iterations  =     12,500
Metropolis-Hastings and Gibbs sampling      Burn-in          =      2,500
                                            MCMC sample size =     10,000
Group variable: neighbourhood               Number of groups =         48

                                            Obs per group:
                                                         min =          4
                                                         avg =       14.3
                                                         max =         49

                                            Number of obs    =        684
                                            Acceptance rate  =      .8101
                                            Efficiency:  min =     .06103
                                                         avg =       .404
Log marginal likelihood                                  max =      .5574
```

	Mean	Std. Dev.	MCSE	Median	Equal-tailed [95% Cred. Interval]	
health						
activity	.5899175	.0380829	.00051	.5898283	.5162173	.6651132
_cons	.7763184	1.938533	.027145	.7782119	-3.043359	4.568399
neighbourhood						
U0:sigma2	4.163866	1.469554	.059484	3.95987	1.907652	7.587148
e.health						
sigma2	29.77787	1.70095	.024359	29.7101	26.65607	33.29967

Note: Default priors are used for model parameters.

information of the simulation procedure to obtain the posterior distribution of the parameters of interest. A detailed explanation of the information given in the first two parts of the output goes beyond the scope of this book. It is important to realise that the prior distributions used in this Bayesian mixed model analysis are the default options in STATA, but they make a lot of sense (Browne and Draper, 2006; Gelwin, 2006).

The last part of both outputs contain the actual results of the analyses. From these results it can be seen that the differences between the two methods are very small. Only the random intercept variance is slightly higher when estimated with a Bayesian mixed model analysis. It is sometimes argued that a Bayesian mixed model analysis is preferable when the number of groups is small and/or the number of subjects within a group is small. To evaluate this, an example is used which is comparable to the example used in Chapter 3, i.e. the dataset from a randomised controlled trial (RCT) to investigate the effect of an intervention to improve health. Health is a continuous outcome variable, and a cluster randomisation was performed among 20 general practitioners (GPs). The randomisation was performed in such a way that for 10 GPs 10 patients were included, and for the other 10 GPs only 2 patients were included. From the 120 patients, 60 received the intervention and 60 did not. Output 13.13 and Output 13.14 show the output of the standard mixed model analysis and the Bayesian mixed model analysis (both with a random intercept on GP level) to investigate the effect of the intervention.

From the results of the two analyses it can be seen that besides the higher random intercept variance, the regression coefficient of the intervention obtained from the Bayesian mixed model analysis is also slightly higher than the one obtained from a standard mixed model analysis. It can also be seen that the 95% credible interval is slightly wider than the 95% confidence interval. However, also in a situation where the number of subjects within the groups is relatively small, there is not much difference between the two methods.

13.3.2 Another Example

Bayesian mixed model analysis can also be used when the outcome variable of interest is dichotomous. The dataset used in the third example of this

Output 13.13 Results of a linear mixed model analysis to determine the effect of the intervention on a continuous health outcome with a random intercept on GP level

```
Mixed-effects ML regression            Number of obs     =        120
Group variable: gp                     Number of groups  =         20

                                       Obs per group:
                                                    min =          2
                                                    avg =        6.0
                                                    max =         10

                                       Wald chi2(1)      =       7.22
Log likelihood = -121.60946            Prob > chi2       =     0.0072

------------------------------------------------------------------------------
      health |    Coef.   Std. Err.      z    P>|z|    [95% Conf. Interval]
-------------+----------------------------------------------------------------
intervention |  .5763604   .2144439    2.69   0.007    .1560581    .9966628
       _cons |  6.475915   .1516348   42.71   0.000    6.178716    6.773113
------------------------------------------------------------------------------


------------------------------------------------------------------------------
  Random-effects Parameters  |   Estimate   Std. Err.    [95% Conf. Interval]
-----------------------------+------------------------------------------------
gp: Identity                 |
                  var(_cons) |   .1402424   .0743242     .0496328    .3962691
-----------------------------+------------------------------------------------
               var(Residual) |    .372327   .0527204      .282096    .4914192
------------------------------------------------------------------------------
LR test vs. linear model: chibar2(01) = 13.29          Prob >= chibar2 = 0.0001
```

section contains data from 40 hospitals in which the risk of dying in the emergency room is investigated. Therefore, over a certain period of time the number of deaths is registered. Out of the 642 patients, 26% died, varying from 0% to 65% for the different hospitals. The number of patients within the different hospitals differed between 5 and 49. An intercept-only mixed model analysis was performed to illustrate the potential use of Bayesian mixed model analyses. Output 13.15 shows the results of the standard logistic mixed model analysis, while Output 13.16 shows the results of the Bayesian logistic mixed model analysis.

From the outputs of both analyses it can be seen that the differences between the results of the standard logistic mixed model analysis and the Bayesian logistic mixed model analysis are comparable to the ones observed for continuous outcomes; a slightly higher regression coefficient, a slightly wider credible interval, and a slightly higher random intercept variance for the Bayesian mixed model analysis. The differences are as expected because

Output 13.14 Results of a Bayesian linear mixed model analysis to determine the effect of the intervention on a continuous health outcome with a random intercept on GP level

```
Multilevel structure
----------------------------------------------------------------------
gp
    {U0}: random intercepts
----------------------------------------------------------------------

Model summary
----------------------------------------------------------------------
Likelihood:
  health ~ normal(xb_health,{e.health:sigma2})

Priors:
  {health:intervention _cons} ~ normal(0,10000)                    (1)
                      {U0} ~ normal(0,{U0:sigma2})                 (1)
          {e.health:sigma2} ~ igamma(.01,.01)

Hyperprior:
  {U0:sigma2} ~ igamma(.01,.01)
----------------------------------------------------------------------
(1) Parameters are elements of the linear form xb_health.


Bayesian multilevel regression           MCMC iterations  =     12,500
Metropolis-Hastings and Gibbs sampling    Burn-in          =      2,500
                                          MCMC sample size =     10,000
Group variable: gp                        Number of groups =         20

                                          Obs per group:
                                                     min =          2
                                                     avg =        6.0
                                                     max =         10

                                          Number of obs   =        120
                                          Acceptance rate =      .8197
                                          Efficiency:  min =    .03035
                                                       avg =     .1061
Log marginal likelihood                                max =     .2854
```

	Mean	Std. Dev.	MCSE	Median	Equal-tailed [95% Cred. Interval]	
health						
intervention	.5930976	.2400761	.013634	.5853143	.1405644	1.1003
_cons	6.466925	.1742254	.01	6.474459	6.09437	6.784391
gp						
U0:sigma2	.1856539	.1072488	.003851	.1623961	.0483803	.4511317
e.health						
sigma2	.3844497	.0588011	.001101	.3789139	.2888922	.5118716

Note: Default priors are used for model parameters.

Output 13.15 Results of an intercept-only logistic mixed model analysis with a random intercept on hospital level

```
Mixed-effects logistic regression          Number of obs     =        642
Group variable:           hospital         Number of groups  =         40

                                           Obs per group:
                                                        min =          5
                                                        avg =       16.1
                                                        max =         49

Integration method: mvaghermite           Integration pts.  =          7

                                          Wald chi2(0)       =          .
Log likelihood = -358.07075               Prob > chi2        =          .
-------------+------------------------------------------------------------
      event |     Coef.   Std. Err.      z    P>|z|    [95% Conf. Interval]
-------------+------------------------------------------------------------
      _cons | -1.152572   .1482664    -7.77   0.000   -1.443169   -.8619754
-------------+------------------------------------------------------------
hospital    |
 var(_cons) |  .4350047   .1874868                     .1869074    1.012422
-------------------------------------------------------------------------
LR test vs. logistic model: chibar2(01) = 19.83     Prob >= chibar2 = 0.0000
```

Output 13.16 Results of an intercept-only Bayesian logistic mixed model analysis with a random intercept on hospital level

```
Multilevel structure
-------------------------------------------------------------------------
hospital
    {U0}: random intercepts
-------------------------------------------------------------------------

Model summary
-------------------------------------------------------------------------
Likelihood:
   event ~ melogit(xb_event)

Priors:
   {event:_cons} ~ normal(0,10000)                                      (1)
          {U0} ~ normal(0,{U0:sigma2})                                  (1)

Hyperprior:
   {U0:sigma2} ~ igamma(.01,.01)
-------------------------------------------------------------------------
(1) Parameters are elements of the linear form xb_event.

Bayesian multilevel logistic regression    MCMC iterations   =     12,500
Random-walk Metropolis-Hastings sampling   Burn-in           =      2,500
                                           MCMC sample size  =     10,000
Group variable: hospital                   Number of groups  =         40

                                           Obs per group:
                                                        min =          5
                                                        avg =       16.1
                                                        max =         49

Family : Bernoulli                         Number of obs     =        642
Link   : logit                             Acceptance rate   =       .379
                                           Efficiency:  min  =     .01793
                                                        avg  =     .02512
Log marginal likelihood                                 max  =     .03231

-------------------------------------------------------------------------
            |                                          Equal-tailed
            |    Mean   Std. Dev.    MCSE    Median  [95% Cred. Interval]
-------------+-----------------------------------------------------------
event       |
      _cons | -1.163113  .1530746  .008516 -1.156374 -1.479437  -.8793217
-------------+-----------------------------------------------------------
hospital    |
  U0:sigma2 |  .4814246  .2170829  .016214   .459149   .145365   .9905062
-------------------------------------------------------------------------
Note: Default priors are used for model parameters.
```

Output 13.17 Probability distribution of the estimated intercepts for each hospital obtained from a Bayesian logistic mixed model analysis

Graphs by parameter

it should be realised that the number of patients and the number of persons that died in some of the hospitals was rather low.

One of the biggest advantages of Bayesian mixed model analysis is the fact that the intercept values for each hospital estimated with the mixed model analysis are not fixed but are derived from a probability distribution. To illustrate this, Output 13.17 shows the distributions of the intercepts for each hospital, while Output 13.18 shows the descriptive information of these distributions for each hospital.

Based on the intercept (-1.163133) and the mean of the variance for each hospital, the probability of dying for each hospital can be calculated. This probability will be more or less the same as the estimated probability derived from a standard logistic mixed model analysis including the random intercept variance (see Chapter 8). However, with a Bayesian approach the risk of dying is not a fixed number, but it is basically a probability distribution (see Output 13.37). With this probability

Output 13.18 Descriptive information of the probability distribution of the estimated intercepts for each hospital obtained from a Bayesian logistic mixed model analysis

```
Bayesian multilevel logistic regression      MCMC iterations  =     12,500
Random-walk Metropolis-Hastings sampling     Burn-in          =      2,500
                                             MCMC sample size =     10,000
Group variable: hospital                     Number of groups =         40

                                             Obs per group:
                                                        min =          5
                                                        avg =       16.1
                                                        max =         49


Family : Bernoulli                           Number of obs    =        642
Link   : logit                               Acceptance rate  =       .379
                                             Efficiency:  min =     .01793
                                                          avg =      .1186
Log marginal likelihood                                   max =      .1879
```

	Mean	Std. Dev.	MCSE	Median	Equal-tailed [95% Cred. Interval]	
event						
_cons	-1.163113	.1530746	.008516	-1.156374	-1.479437	-.8793217
U0[hospital]						
1	-.1313943	.4070194	.012348	-.1297207	-.9766654	.6565067
2	-.074939	.5193935	.012927	-.053583	-1.159881	.9154703
3	-.4919918	.6320502	.016508	-.4461279	-1.86818	.6389596
4	-.9567359	.5468916	.021117	-.9266463	-2.158372	-.018731
5	1.06033	.4414224	.022192	1.034129	.2491874	1.951928
6	-.6570064	.5767517	.017033	-.5876658	-1.919741	.3574019
7	.2941016	.4912418	.01368	.2857642	-.6418836	1.254263
8	-.6141629	.4680625	.01556	-.5951772	-1.591427	.2299249
9	1.128797	.45781	.022886	1.126679	.2572846	2.060064
10	.3544813	.5041521	.014249	.3655144	-.6262681	1.356863
11	.0102987	.4507516	.011496	.0121026	-.9174023	.8967641
12	-.280385	.4880208	.01181	-.2575543	-1.290362	.6150575
13	.1544097	.4034295	.011423	.1465412	-.6556719	.9556516
14	.2224096	.5780695	.014642	.2123193	-.8862904	1.388934
15	-.5282418	.5315996	.014104	-.5006757	-1.676098	.4382479
16	.4198504	.3187731	.012594	.4174362	-.2051058	1.056671
17	.0238503	.4774459	.012583	.0274545	-.9566769	.945711
18	-.3451059	.5432004	.013832	-.3255287	-1.531137	.6562484
19	.0859316	.525514	.012124	.0966684	-.954615	1.066795
20	-.3387197	.4538292	.011384	-.3339984	-1.318701	.504622
21	.0699309	.4911424	.012916	.0728676	-.9034425	1.018169
22	-.129329	.4614999	.011732	-.1370245	-1.062937	.7632165
23	-.142394	.477468	.011926	-.1409336	-1.178966	.7510221
24	-.4977502	.4841726	.014262	-.4666867	-1.486521	.382427
25	-.1806266	.4972916	.012465	-.175369	-1.184908	.7934218
26	.2587093	.4473995	.013387	.254584	-.6410756	1.151908
27	.1353172	.4988931	.012869	.134575	-.8619228	1.119126
28	-.1205169	.509421	.012802	-.1172101	-1.152762	.8596868
29	.2876619	.4084309	.012923	.2895117	-.4914972	1.103015
30	.8605599	.4103914	.021059	.8583464	.0814545	1.707414
31	.376765	.4377599	.01297	.3749854	-.4768076	1.268953
32	-.3310936	.4402389	.012567	-.3142427	-1.244698	.4609064
33	.390471	.4072572	.013514	.385916	-.4035193	1.189722
34	.8360243	.4462536	.021934	.8211739	-.0187498	1.768452
35	.1338356	.414137	.011883	.1244501	-.6808561	.9146897
36	.0081781	.490512	.012399	.0194331	-1.013844	.9544403
37	-.1021701	.4758519	.011961	-.081585	-1.106083	.8014078
38	.0193852	.4898336	.012541	.0382827	-.9968969	.968005
39	-1.122219	.4995623	.021623	-1.083918	-2.176146	-.2691636
40	.125926	.4845046	.01262	.1249991	-.8450667	1.109992
hospital						
U0:sigma2	.4814246	.2170829	.016214	.459149	.145365	.9905062

Note: Default priors are used for model parameters.

distribution it is possible to answer more detailed research questions regarding the comparison between hospitals. For instance, it will be possible to estimate the probability that the risk of dying in one hospital is bigger than the risk of dying in another hospital.

13.3.3 Comments

The biggest advantage of Bayesian mixed model analysis is that prior information can be used for the estimation of effects. However, when no detailed prior information is available in a particular situation, the advantage of Bayesian mixed model analyses is rather limited. Besides that, adding the appropriate prior information to the analysis is a very difficult procedure.

As has been shown in Section 13.3.1, in some situations specific research questions can be answered with a Bayesian mixed model analysis that cannot be answered with a standard mixed model analysis. This has mostly to do with the fact that the estimated parameters are not fixed but are based on a probability distribution. Therefore, the 95% credible interval obtained from a Bayesian mixed model analysis has a more straightforward interpretation compared to the 95% confidence interval obtained from a standard mixed model analysis. Therefore, it is possible, for instance, to estimate the probability that one group is better or worse than another group, etc.

The reason for writing this section is that Bayesian mixed model analysis has gained popularity over the last few years. However, it should be realised that Bayesian mixed model analysis is very complicated. The examples shown in this chapter are relatively simple, using default priors for the Bayesian mixed model analysis. Using Bayesian analysis requires knowledge about the basic mathematics of probability distributions, and the choices that can be made regarding priors are numerous and often difficult to make.

13.4 Software

13.4.1 Introduction

In the foregoing chapters all examples of mixed model analyses were analysed with STATA. Although STATA is widely used and perfectly suitable for mixed model analyses, mixed model analyses can also be performed with other software programs such as SAS, SPSS and R. In Section 13.4.3 the results of mixed model analyses performed with other software programs will be presented. First, in Section 13.4.2, the syntax that was used for the examples in the foregoing chapters is shown.

13.4.2 STATA Syntax

For readers who want to reanalyse the data of the different examples, Table 13.2 (linear mixed model analysis), Table 13.3 (logistic, multinomial

Table 13.2 Syntax used to perform linear mixed model analysis with STATA

Linear (intercept only) mixed model analysis with two levels with random intercept:
```
mixed health || neighbourhood:
```
Linear mixed model analysis with two levels with random intercept:
```
mixed health activity || neighbourhood:
```
Linear mixed model analysis with two levels with random intercept and random slope and an unstructured covariance structure:
```
mixed health activity || neighbourhood: activity, cov(unstruct)
```
Linear mixed model analysis with three levels and random intercept on both levels:
```
mixed health activity || region: || neighbourhood:
```

Table 13.3 Syntax used to perform different logistic mixed model analyses with STATA

Logistic mixed model analysis with two levels with random intercept:
```
melogit health_dich activity || neighbourhood:
```
Ordinal logistic mixed model analysis with two levels with random intercept:
```
meologit health_cat activity || neighbourhood:
```
Multinomial logistic regression analysis with two levels with random intercept (performed with the gllamm procedure in STATA):
```
gen cons = 1
eq cons: cons
gllamm health_cat activity, link(mlogit) fam(binom)
  i(neighbourhood)
```
Multinomial logistic regression analysis with two levels with random intercept and random slope (performed with the gllamm procedure in STATA)
```
gen cons = 1
eq cons: cons
eq act: activity
gllamm health_cat activity, link(mlogit) fam(binom)
  i(neighbourhood) nrf(2) eqs(cons act)
```

Table 13.4 Syntax used to perform Poisson mixed model analyses with STATA

Poisson mixed model analysis with two levels with random intercept:
```
mepoisson falls age || home:
```
Negative binomial mixed model analysis with two levels with random intercept:
```
menbreg falls age || home:
```

Table 13.5 Syntax used to perform parametric survival mixed model analyses with STATA

Exponential survival mixed model analysis with two levels with random intercept:
```
stset follow_up, failure(recovery)
mestreg treatment || therapist:, dist(exponential)
```
Weibull survival mixed model analysis with two levels with random intercept:
```
stset follow_up, failure(recovery)
mestreg treatment || therapist:, dist(weibull)
```

---

logistic and ordered logistic mixed model analysis), Table 13.4 (Poisson and negative binomial mixed model analysis) and Table 13.5 (mixed survival analysis) show the syntax used to perform the mixed model analyses on the example datasets, which results were shown in the foregoing chapters.

13.4.3 Other Software

As has been mentioned before, mixed model analyses can also be performed with other software programs such as SAS, SPSS and R. To illustrate the use of these programs, a few examples of the foregoing chapters will be reanalysed in this section with other software programs.

13.4.3.1 Linear Mixed Model Analysis with Two Levels

Firstly, the examples of Chapter 2 in which the relationship between physical activity and health was analysed will be reanalysed. Output 13.19 shows the result of the mixed model analysis performed with STATA; this output was already shown in Output 2.3. Output 13.20, Output 13.21 and

Output 13.19 Result of a linear mixed model analysis of the relationship between physical activity and health, with a random intercept on neighbourhood level performed with STATA

```
Mixed-effects ML regression            Number of obs     =        684
Group variable: neighbourhood          Number of groups  =         48

                                       Obs per group:
                                                    min =          4
                                                    avg =       14.3
                                                    max =         49

                                       Wald chi2(1)      =     241.50
Log likelihood = -2153.4088            Prob > chi2       =     0.0000

------------------------------------------------------------------------------
    health |    Coef.   Std. Err.      z    P>|z|     [95% Conf. Interval]
-----------+------------------------------------------------------------------
  activity |  .5896818   .037945    15.54   0.000     .515311    .6640527
     _cons |  .7898844  1.941018     0.41   0.684    -3.01444    4.594209
------------------------------------------------------------------------------


------------------------------------------------------------------------------
  Random-effects Parameters  |   Estimate   Std. Err.    [95% Conf. Interval]
-----------------------------+------------------------------------------------
neighbourhood: Identity      |
                var(_cons)   |  4.018727   1.359694     2.070587    7.799802
-----------------------------+------------------------------------------------
               var(Residual) |  29.57958   1.661547    26.49587    33.02218
------------------------------------------------------------------------------
LR test vs. linear model: chibar2(01) = 30.96         Prob >= chibar2 = 0.0000
```

Output 13.22 show the results of the same analyses performed with SPSS, R and SAS respectively.

Comparing the different software programs with each other, it should be noted that within SAS, SPSS and R the restricted maximum likelihood is the default estimation procedure (see Section 2.8.3). From the outputs it can further be seen that SAS, SPSS and R use the t-distribution to obtain the 95% confidence intervals around the regression coefficients and to obtain the p-value, whereas STATA uses the standard normal distribution. However, with the number of degrees of freedom (related to the number of observations) in the present example, the t-distribution and the standard normal distribution are almost the same, so the difference between the two is very small.

Table 13.6 provides an overview of the results obtained from the different software programs.

From Table 13.6 it can be seen that the results of the linear mixed model analyses of the relationship between physical activity and health with only a

Output 13.20 Syntax and result of a mixed model analysis of the relationship between physical activity and health, with a random intercept on neighbourhood level performed with SPSS

```
MIXED health WITH activity

  /CRITERIA=CIN(95) MXITER(100) MXSTEP(10) SCORING(1)
SINGULAR(0.000000000001) HCONVERGE(0, ABSOLUTE) LCONVERGE(0,
ABSOLUTE) PCONVERGE(0.000001, ABSOLUTE)

  /FIXED=activity | SSTYPE(3)

  /METHOD=REML

  /PRINT=SOLUTION

  /RANDOM=INTERCEPT | SUBJECT(neigbourhood) COVTYPE(VC).
```

Information criteria[a]

−2 restricted log likelihood	4311.675
Akaike's information criterion (AIC)	4315.675
Hurvich and Tsai's criterion (AICC)	4315.692
Bozdogan's criterion (CAIC)	4326.725
Schwarz's Bayesian criterion (BIC)	4324.725

The information criteria are displayed in smaller-is-better form

[a] Dependent variable: health.

Estimates of fixed effects[a]

						95% confidence interval	
Parameter	Estimate	Std. Error	df	t	Sig.	Lower bound	Upper bound
Intercept	0.792191	1.944459	673.636	0.407	0.684	−3.025738	4.610120
Activity	0.589640	0.037997	681.016	15.518	0.000	0.515035	0.664244

[a] Dependent variable: health.

Estimates of covariance parameters[a]

Parameter		Estimate	Std. error
Residual		29.619668	1.664813
Intercept [subject = neigbourhood]	Variance	4.172779	1.408115

[a] Dependent variable: health.

Output 13.21 Syntax and result of a mixed model analysis of the relationship between physical activity and health, with a random intercept on neighbourhood level performed with R

```
out <- lme(health ~ activity, random = ~ 1|neigbourhood, method="ML",
data=dataset)
```

```
Linear mixed-effects model fit by maximum likelihood
 Data: data
       AIC       BIC     logLik
  4314.818 4332.929 -2153.409

Random effects:
 Formula: ~1 | neighbourhood
         (Intercept) Residual
StdDev:    2.004692 5.438709

Fixed effects: health ~ activity
                 Value Std.Error  DF   t-value p-value
(Intercept) 0.7898855 1.9438619 635  0.406349  0.6846
activity    0.5896818 0.0380006 635 15.517691  0.0000
 Correlation:
          (Intr)
activity -0.982

Standardized Within-Group Residuals:
       Min         Q1        Med        Q3        Max
-3.8450937 -0.5622782  0.1365826  0.6346987  2.7226033

Number of Observations: 684
Number of Groups: 48
```

random intercept on neighbourhood level are very stable. The regression coefficients, corresponding standard errors and the random intercept variances are the same.

13.4.3.2 Linear Mixed Model Analysis with Two Levels Including a Random Slope

Secondly, the examples of Chapter 2 in which the relationship between physical activity and health was analysed with both a random intercept and random slope for physical activity will be reanalysed. To avoid convergence problems, the analyses were performed using the centred value for physical activity (see Section 2.5). Output 13.23 shows the result of the mixed model analysis performed with STATA; this output was already shown in Output 2.7. Output 13.24, Output 13.25 and Output 13.26 show the results of the same analyses performed with SPSS, R and SAS respectively.

Output 13.22 Syntax and results of a mixed model analysis of the relationship between physical activity and health, with a random intercept on neighbourhood level performed with SAS

```
PROC MIXED data = cont method=ml;
class neighbourhood;
model health = activity/s;
random int /subject=neighbourhood type=vc;
RUN;
```

Fit Statistics	
-2 Log Likelihood	4306.8
AIC (Smaller is Better)	4314.8
AICC (Smaller is Better)	4314.9
BIC (Smaller is Better)	4322.3

Solution for Fixed Effects					
Effect	Estimate	Standard Error	DF	t Value	Pr > |t|
Intercept	0.7899	1.9410	47	0.41	0.6859
activity	0.5897	0.03795	635	15.54	<.0001

Covariance Parameter Estimates		
Cov Parm	Subject	Estimate
UN(1,1)	neighbourhood	4.0179
Residual		29.5799

Table 13.6 Overview of the results of a linear mixed model analysis of the relationship between physical activity and health, with a random intercept on neighbourhood level estimated with different software packages

	Regression coefficient (SE)	Random variance intercept
STATA	0.5897 (0.0379)	4.019
SPSS	0.5897 (0.0379)	4.019
R	0.5897 (0.0380)	4.019
SAS	0.5897 (0.0380)	4.018

Output 13.23 Result of a linear mixed model analysis of the relationship between physical activity (centred) and health, with both a random intercept and a random slope for activity on neighbourhood level performed with STATA

```
Mixed-effects ML regression                    Number of obs    =       684
Group variable: neighbourhood                  Number of groups =        48

                                               Obs per group:
                                                            min =         4
                                                            avg =      14.3
                                                            max =        49

                                               Wald chi2(1)     =    143.45
Log likelihood = -2142.4879                    Prob > chi2      =    0.0000

-----------------------------------------------------------------------------
     health |     Coef.   Std. Err.      z    P>|z|    [95% Conf. Interval]
------------+----------------------------------------------------------------
 activity_c~t |  .5901689   .0492746   11.98   0.000    .4935925    .6867453
       _cons |  30.37344   .3928229   77.32   0.000    29.60352    31.14336
-----------------------------------------------------------------------------


-----------------------------------------------------------------------------
  Random-effects Parameters  |   Estimate   Std. Err.    [95% Conf. Interval]
-----------------------------+-----------------------------------------------
neighbourhood: Unstructured  |
              var(activi~t)  |   .0455241   .0233207      .01668    .1242473
                var(_cons)   |   4.958736   1.551291    2.685846    9.155051
         cov(activi~t,_cons) |  -.467691    .1567888    -.7749914   -.1603905
-----------------------------+-----------------------------------------------
                var(Residual)|   27.98527   1.614951    24.99246    31.33646
-----------------------------------------------------------------------------
LR test vs. linear model: chi2(3) = 52.80               Prob > chi2 = 0.0000
```

Table 13.7 provides an overview of the results obtained from the different software programs.

From Table 13.7 it can be seen that the linear mixed model analyses with both a random intercept and a random slope for physical activity on the neighbourhood level are very stable too. The regression coefficients, standard errors, random intercept variance, random slope variance, and covariance between random intercept and random slope are the same for all programs.

13.4.3.3 Linear Mixed Model Analysis with Three Levels

Thirdly, the examples of Chapter 2 in which the relationship between physical activity and health was analysed with a random intercept on neighbourhood level and a random intercept on region level will be reanalysed. Output 13.27 shows the result of the mixed model analysis performed with STATA; this output was already shown in Qutput 2.8. Output 13.28,

Output 13.24 Syntax and result of a linear mixed model analysis of the relationship between physical activity (centred) and health, with both a random intercept and a random slope for activity on neighbourhood level performed with SPSS

```
MIXED health WITH activity_cent
   /CRITERIA=CIN(95) MXITER(100) MXSTEP(10) SCORING(1)
SINGULAR(0.000000000001) HCONVERGE(0, ABSOLUTE) LCONVERGE(0,
ABSOLUTE) PCONVERGE(0.000001, ABSOLUTE)
   /FIXED=activity_cent | SSTYPE(3)
   /METHOD=ML
   /PRINT=SOLUTION
   /RANDOM=INTERCEPT activity_cent | SUBJECT(neighbourhood)
COVTYPE(UN).
```

Information criteria[a]

−2 log likelihood	4284.976
Akaike's Information criterion (AIC)	4296.976
Hurvich and Tsai's criterion (AICC)	4297.100
Bozdogan's criterion (CAIC)	4330.144
Schwarz's Bayesian criterion (BIC)	4324.144

The information criteria are displayed in smaller-is-better form

[a] Dependent variable: health.

Estimates of fixed effects[a]

						95% confidence interval	
Parameter	Estimate	Std. error	df	t	Sig.	Lower bound	Upper bound
Intercept	30.373439	0.392823	43.107	77.321	0.000	29.581292	31.165586
activity_cent	0.590168	0.049273	39.608	11.978	0.000	0.490553	0.689783

[a] Dependent variable: health.

Estimates of covariance parameters[a]

Parameter		Estimate	Std. error
Residual		27.985478	1.615434
Intercept + activity_cent [subject = neighbourhood]	UN (1.1)	4.958771	1.551315
	UN (2.1)	−0.467700	0.156855
	UN (2.2)	0.045517	0.023348

[a] Dependent variable: health.

Output 13.25 Syntax and result of a linear mixed model analysis of the relationship between physical activity (centred) and health, with both a random intercept and a random slope for activity on neighbourhood level performed with R

```
> out1 <- lme(health ~ activity_cent, random = ~
activity_cent|neighbourhood, method="ML", data=data)
```

```
Linear mixed-effects model fit by maximum likelihood
 Data: data
      AIC      BIC   logLik
  4296.976 4324.144 -2142.488

Random effects:
 Formula: ~activity_cent | neighbourhood
 Structure: General positive-definite, Log-Cholesky parametrization
               StdDev    Corr
(Intercept)   2.2268054 (Intr)
activity_cent 0.2133501 -0.984
Residual      5.2901265

Fixed effects: health ~ activity_cent
                 Value Std.Error  DF  t-value p-value
(Intercept)   30.373439 0.3933960 635 77.20830       0
activity_cent  0.590168 0.0493453 635 11.95996       0
 Correlation:
               (Intr)
activity_cent -0.566

Standardized Within-Group Residuals:
      Min         Q1        Med        Q3        Max
 -3.9751124 -0.5310949  0.1513124  0.6392860  2.5850382

Number of Observations: 684
Number of Groups: 48
```

Output 13.29 and Output 13.30 show the results of the same analyses performed with SPSS, R and SAS respectively.

Table 13.8 provides an overview of the results obtained from the different software programs.

Unsurprisingly, from Table 13.8 it can be seen that for the linear mixed model analysis with a three level structure the results are very stable as well. The regression coefficients, standard errors and the random intercept variances at both levels are the same for the four software programs.

Output 13.26 Syntax and result of a linear mixed model analysis of the relationship between physical activity (centred) and health, with both a random intercept and a random slope for activity on neighbourhood level performed with SAS

```
PROC MIXED data = cont method=ml;
class neighbourhood;
model health = activity_cent/s;
random int activity_cent / subject=neighbourhood type=un;
RUN;
```

Fit Statistics	
-2 Log Likelihood	4285.0
AIC (Smaller is Better)	4297.0
AICC (Smaller is Better)	4297.1
BIC (Smaller is Better)	4308.2

Solution for Fixed Effects					
Effect	Estimate	Standard Error	DF	t Value	Pr > |t|
Intercept	30.3734	0.3928	47	77.33	<.0001
activity_cent	0.5902	0.04927	47	11.98	<.0001

Covariance Parameter Estimates			
Cov Parm	Subject	Estimate	Standard Error
UN(1,1)	neighbourhood	0.5020	0.2269
UN(2,1)	neighbourhood	-0.01662	0.01887
UN(2,2)	neighbourhood	0.000825	0.003406

Table 13.7 Overview of the results of a linear mixed model analysis of the relationship between physical activity (centred) and health, with a random intercept and random slope for activity on neighbourhood level estimated with different software packages

	Regression coefficient (SE)	Random variance		
		Intercept	Activity	Covariance
STATA	0.5902 (0.0493)	4.959	0.046	−0.468
SPSS	0.5902 (0.0493)	4.959	0.046	−0.468
R	0.5902 (0.0493)	4.959	0.046	−0.984*
SAS	0.5902 (0.0493)	4.958	0.046	−0.468

* R provides the correlation between random intercept and random slope instead of covariance.

Output 13.27 Result of a linear mixed model analysis of the relationship between physical activity and health, with a random intercept on neighbourhood level and a random intercept on region level performed with STATA

```
Mixed-effects ML regression                      Number of obs    =      684

-----------------------------------------------------------------------------
                     |  No. of      Observations per Group
  Group Variable |  Groups    Minimum    Average    Maximum
---------------------+-------------------------------------------------------
          region |      12         22        57.0         84
    neighbourh~d |      48          4        14.3         49
-----------------------------------------------------------------------------

                                            Wald chi2(1)     =     236.16
Log likelihood = -2146.8629                 Prob > chi2      =     0.0000

-----------------------------------------------------------------------------
      health |    Coef.    Std. Err.      z    P>|z|    [95% Conf. Interval]
-------------+---------------------------------------------------------------
    activity |  .579524    .0377111    15.37   0.000    .5056115    .6534364
       _cons |   1.4913    1.980434     0.75   0.451   -2.390279    5.372879
-----------------------------------------------------------------------------


-----------------------------------------------------------------------------
  Random-effects Parameters  |   Estimate   Std. Err.    [95% Conf. Interval]
-----------------------------+-----------------------------------------------
region: Identity             |
                var(_cons)   |  2.947866   1.569788     1.038075    8.371184
-----------------------------+-----------------------------------------------
neighbourh~d: Identity       |
                var(_cons)   |  1.128718   .7955629      .2835481    4.493081
-----------------------------+-----------------------------------------------
             var(Residual)   |  29.50382    1.65266      26.43615    32.92748
-----------------------------------------------------------------------------
LR test vs. linear model: chi2(2) = 44.05            Prob > chi2 = 0.0000
```

13.4.3.4 Logistic Mixed Model Analysis with Two Levels

Fourthly, the examples of Chapter 4 in which the relationship between physical activity and the dichotomous health indicator was analysed with a random intercept on neighbourhood level will be reanalysed. Output 13.31 shows the result of the logistic mixed model analysis performed with STATA; this output was already shown in Output 4.3. Output 13.32, Output 13.33 and Output 13.34 show the results of the same analyses performed with SPSS, R and SAS respectively.

From the syntaxes used in the different programs, it can be seen that different procedures must be applied for logistic mixed model analysis than for linear mixed model analysis. For linear mixed model analysis in SPSS and SAS the procedure MIXED can be used, while in R the procedure lme

Output 13.28 Syntax and result of a linear mixed model analysis of the relationship between physical activity and health, with a random intercept on neighbourhood level and a random intercept on region level performed with SPSS

```
MIXED health WITH activity
  /CRITERIA=CIN(95) MXITER(100) MXSTEP(10) SCORING(1)
SINGULAR(0.000000000001) HCONVERGE(0, ABSOLUTE) LCONVERGE(0,
ABSOLUTE) PCONVERGE(0.000001, ABSOLUTE)
  /FIXED=activity | SSTYPE(3)
  /METHOD=ML
  /PRINT=SOLUTION
  /RANDOM=INTERCEPT | SUBJECT(neighbourhood) COVTYPE(VC)
  /RANDOM=INTERCEPT | SUBJECT(region) COVTYPE(VC)
```

Information criteria[a]

−2 log likelihood	4293.726
Akaike's Information criterion (AIC)	4303.726
Hurvich and Tsai's criterion (AICC)	4303.814
Bozdogan's criterion (CAIC)	4331.366
Schwarz's Bayesian criterion (BIC)	4326.366

The information criteria are displayed in smaller-is-better form.

[a] Dependent variable: health.

Estimates of fixed effects[a]

Parameter	Estimate	Std. error	df	t	Sig.	95% confidence interval	
						Lower bound	Upper bound
Intercept	1.491298	1.980433	505.061	0.753	0.452	−2.399604	5.382200
	0.579524	0.037711	682.798	15.367	0.000	0.505480	0.653568

[a] Dependent variable: health.

Estimates of covariance parameters[a]

Parameter		Estimate	Std. error
Residual		29.503826	1.652661
Intercept [subject = neihgbourhood]	Variance	1.128720	0.795566
Intercept [subject = region]	Variance	2.947837	1.569771

[a] Dependent variable: health.

Output 13.29 Syntax and result of a linear mixed model analysis of the relationship between physical activity and health, with a random intercept on neighbourhood level and a random intercept on region level performed with R

```
> out <- lme(health ~ activity, random = ~1|region/neighbourhood,
method="ML", data=data)
```

```
Linear mixed-effects model fit by maximum likelihood
 Data: data
       AIC      BIC     logLik
  4303.726 4326.366 -2146.863

Random effects:
 Formula: ~1 | region
         (Intercept)
StdDev:    1.716928

 Formula: ~1 | neighbourhood %in% region
         (Intercept) Residual
StdDev:    1.062406 5.431743

Fixed effects: health ~ activity
               Value Std.Error  DF   t-value p-value
(Intercept) 1.491300 1.9833348 635  0.751916  0.4524
activity    0.579524 0.0377664 635 15.344963  0.0000
 Correlation:
          (Intr)
activity -0.958

Standardized Within-Group Residuals:
       Min         Q1        Med        Q3        Max
-4.0357426 -0.5692696  0.1393110  0.6202332  2.7035607

Number of Observations: 684
Number of Groups:
                    region neighbourhood %in% region
                        12                        48
```

---

was used. For logistic mixed model analysis the procedures GENLIN-MIXED (SPSS), glmer(R) and GLIMMIX (SAS) can be used. It should be noted that for R (glmmPQL) and SAS (NLMIXED) other procedures can also be used to estimate the coefficients of a logistic mixed model analysis.

Output 13.30 Syntax and result of a linear mixed model analysis of the relationship between physical activity and health, with a random intercept on neighbourhood level and a random intercept on region level performed with SAS

```
PROC MIXED data = cont method=ml;
class neighbourhood region;
model health = activity/s;
random int / subject=neighbourhood type=un;
random int / subject=region type=un;
RUN;
```

Fit Statistics	
-2 Log Likelihood	4293.7
AIC (Smaller is Better)	4303.7
AICC (Smaller is Better)	4303.8
BIC (Smaller is Better)	4293.7

Solution for Fixed Effects					
Effect	Estimate	Standard Error	DF	t Value	Pr > |t|
Intercept	1.4913	1.9804	0	0.75	.
activity	0.5795	0.03771	635	15.37	<.0001

Covariance Parameter Estimates		
Cov Parm	Subject	Estimate
UN(1,1)	neighbourhood	1.1287
UN(1,1)	region	2.9478
Residual		29.5038

Table 13.8 Overview of the results of a linear mixed model analysis of the relationship between physical activity and health, with a random intercept on neighbourhood level and a random intercept on region level estimated with different software packages

	Regression coefficient (SE)	Random variance intercept	
		Neighbourhood	Region
STATA	0.5795 (0.0377)	1.129	2.948
SPSS	0.5795 (0.0377)	1.129	2.948
R	0.5795 (0.0378)	1.129	2.948
SAS	0.5795 (0.0377)	1.129	2.948

Output 13.31 Result of a logistic mixed model analysis of the relationship between physical activity and the dichotomous health indicator with a random intercept on neighbourhood level performed with STATA

```
Mixed-effects logistic regression           Number of obs     =        684
Group variable:     neighbourhood           Number of groups  =         48

                                            Obs per group:
                                                         min =          4
                                                         avg =       14.3
                                                         max =         49

Integration method: mvaghermite             Integration pts.  =          7

                                            Wald chi2(1)      =      83.43
Log likelihood = -408.96783                 Prob > chi2       =     0.0000
-------------------------------------------------------------------------
  health_dich |   Coef.   Std. Err.     z    P>|z|   [95% Conf. Interval]
--------------+----------------------------------------------------------
     activity |  .1685528  .0184534    9.13  0.000   .1323849   .2047207
        _cons | -8.243316  .9319357   -8.85  0.000  -10.06988  -6.416756
--------------+----------------------------------------------------------
neighbourhood |
    var(_cons)|  .4866812  .2171715           .2029613   1.167013
-------------------------------------------------------------------------
LR test vs. logistic model: chibar2(01) = 16.60      Prob >= chibar2 = 0.0000
```

Table 13.9 provides an overview of the results obtained from the different software programs.

From Table 13.9 it can be seen that logistic mixed model analyses with only a random intercept are not as stable as the linear mixed model analyses. Regarding the regression coefficients and standard errors, SPSS especially gives different results compared to STATA, R and SAS. This also

Output 13.32 Syntax and result of a logistic mixed model analysis of the relationship between physical activity and the dichotomous health indicator with a random intercept on neighbourhood level performed with SPSS

```
GENLINMIXED
    /DATA_STRUCTURE SUBJECTS=neigbourhood
    /FIELDS TARGET=health_dich TRIALS=NONE OFFSET=NONE
    /TARGET_OPTIONS DISTRIBUTION=BINOMIAL LINK=LOGIT
    /FIXED  EFFECTS=activity USE_INTERCEPT=TRUE
    /RANDOM USE_INTERCEPT=TRUE SUBJECTS=neighbourhood
COVARIANCE_TYPE=VARIANCE_COMPONENTS
    /BUILD_OPTIONS TARGET_CATEGORY_ORDER=DESCENDING
INPUTS_CATEGORY_ORDER=DESCENDING MAX_ITERATIONS=100
CONFIDENCE_LEVEL=95 DF_METHOD=RESIDUAL COVB=MODEL
PCONVERGE=0.000001(ABSOLUTE) SCORING=0 SINGULAR=0.000000000001
    /EMMEANS_OPTIONS SCALE=ORIGINAL PADJUST=LSD.
```

Model summary

Target		health_dich
Probability distribution		Binomial
Link function		Logit
Information criterion	Akaike corrected	3065.074
	Bayesian	3069.594

Information criteria are based on the −2 log likelihood (3063.069) and are used to compare models. Models with smaller information criterion values fit better.

Fixed coefficients[a]

Model term	Coefficient	Std. error	t	Sig.	95% confidence interval	
					Lower	Upper
Intercept	−7.903	0.8908	−8.872	0.000	−9.652	−6.154
Activity	0.162	0.0176	9.187	0.000	0.127	0.196

Probability distribution: binomial

Link function: Logit

[a] Target: health_dich

Random effect

Random effect covariance	Estimate	Std. error	Z	Sig.	95% confidence interval	
					Lower	Upper
Var (intercept)	0.443	0.190	2.328	0.020	0.191	1.029

Covariance structure: variance components

Subject specification: neighbourhood

Output 13.33 Syntax and result of a logistic mixed model analysis of the relationship between physical activity and the dichotomous health indicator with a random intercept on neighbourhood level performed with R

```
> out <- glmer(health_dich ~ activity + (1|neighbourhood), data=data,
family=binomial)
```

```
Generalized linear mixed model fit by maximum likelihood (Laplace
Approximation) ['glmerMod']
 Family: binomial  ( logit )
Formula: health_dich ~ activity + (1 | neighbourhood)
   Data: data

    AIC      BIC   logLik deviance df.resid
  824.3    837.9   -409.2    818.3      681

Scaled residuals:
    Min      1Q  Median      3Q     Max
-3.2845 -0.8172  0.3647  0.7161  3.2790

Random effects:
 Groups        Name         Variance Std.Dev.
 neighbourhood (Intercept) 0.4701    0.6857
Number of obs: 684, groups:  neighbourhood, 48

Fixed effects:
            Estimate Std. Error z value Pr(>|z|)
(Intercept) -8.23870    0.92957  -8.863   <2e-16 ***
activity     0.16845    0.01841   9.152   <2e-16 ***
---
Signif. codes:  0 '***' 0.001 '**' 0.01 '*' 0.05 '.' 0.1 ' ' 1

Correlation of Fixed Effects:
        (Intr)
activity -0.989
```

applies, more or less, for the random intercept variance, although the random intercept variance estimated with STATA is also slightly different from the random intercept variance estimated with R and SAS.

13.4.3.5 Logistic Mixed Model Analysis with Two Levels Including a Random Slope

Finally, the examples of Chapter 4 in which the relationship between physical activity and the dichotomous health indicator was analysed with a random intercept and a random slope for activity on neighbourhood level will be reanalysed. Just as for the same analysis with a continuous outcome (see Section 13.4.3.2), for the logistic mixed model analysis these analyses

Output 13.34 Syntax and result of a logistic mixed model analysis of the relationship between physical activity and the dichotomous health indicator with a random intercept on neighbourhood level performed with SAS

```
PROC GLIMMIX data = dich method=LAPLACE;
class neighbourhood;
model health_dich = activity/s dist=binomial;
random int / subject=neighbourhood type=un;
RUN;
```

Fit Statistics	
-2 Log Likelihood	818.32
AIC (smaller is better)	824.32
AICC (smaller is better)	824.35
BIC (smaller is better)	829.93
CAIC (smaller is better)	832.93
HQIC (smaller is better)	826.44

Solutions for Fixed Effects					
Effect	Estimate	Standard Error	DF	t Value	Pr > |t|
Intercept	-8.2395	0.9311	47	-8.85	<.0001
activity	0.1685	0.01844	635	9.14	<.0001

Covariance Parameter Estimates			
Cov Parm	Subject	Estimate	Standard Error
UN(1,1)	neighbourhood	0.4704	0.2109

Table 13.9 Overview of results of a logistic mixed model analyses of the relationship between physical activity and the dichotomous health indicator with a random intercept on neighbourhood level estimated with different software packages

	Regression coefficient (SE)	Random variance intercept
STATA	0.1686 (0.0185)	0.4867
SPSS	0.1620 (0.0176)	0.443
R	0.1685 (0.0184)	0.4701
SAS	0.1685 (0.0184)	0.4704

Output 13.35 Result of a logistic mixed model analysis of the relationship between physical activity (centred) and the dichotomous health indicator with a random intercept and random slope for activity on neighbourhood level performed with STATA

```
Mixed-effects logistic regression          Number of obs    =       684
Group variable:    neighbourhood           Number of groups =        48

                                           Obs per group:
                                                        min =         4
                                                        avg =      14.3
                                                        max =        49

Integration method: mvaghermite            Integration pts. =         7

                                           Wald chi2(1)     =     68.57
Log likelihood = -408.45993                Prob > chi2      =    0.0000
---------------------------------------------------------------------------
    health_dich |    Coef.   Std. Err.     z    P>|z|   [95% Conf. Interval]
----------------+----------------------------------------------------------
  activity_cent |  .171361   .0206947    8.28   0.000    .1308002    .2119218
          _cons |  .1893429  .1437217    1.32   0.188   -.0923465    .4710323
----------------+----------------------------------------------------------
neighbourhood   |
var(activity_cent)| .0010688 .0035978                    1.46e-06    .7837082
     var(_cons) |  .5191823  .2332014                     .2152709   1.252145
----------------+----------------------------------------------------------
neighbourhood   |
cov(_cons,activity_cent)| -.0176314 .0197326 -0.89 0.372 -.0563066    .0210438
---------------------------------------------------------------------------
LR test vs. logistic model: chi2(3) = 17.62          Prob > chi2 = 0.0005
```

were also performed using the centred value for physical activity. Again, this is done to avoid convergence problems. Output 13.35 shows the result of the logistic mixed model analysis performed with STATA; this output was already shown in Output 4.5. Output 13.36, Output 13.37 and Output 13.38 show the results of the same analyses performed with SPSS, R and SAS respectively.

Table 13.10 provides an overview of the results obtained from the different software programs.

From Table 13.10 it can be seen that the logistic mixed model analyses with both a random intercept and a random slope for activity on neighbourhood level are not very stable either. There is a difference in regression coefficients, standard errors and random variances between the different software programs.

It should be noted that the logistic mixed model analyses were performed with different estimation procedures which obviously lead to slightly different results. Because it is not clear which of the estimation procedures is the most valid, it is hard to give advice about which of the programs to use.

Output 13.36 Syntax and result of a logistic mixed model analysis of the relationship between physical activity and the dichotomous health indicator with a random intercept and random slope for activity on neighbourhood level performed with SPSS

```
GENLINMIXED
  /DATA_STRUCTURE SUBJECTS=neigbourhood
  /FIELDS TARGET=health_dich TRIALS=NONE OFFSET=NONE
  /TARGET_OPTIONS DISTRIBUTION=BINOMIAL LINK=LOGIT
  /FIXED  EFFECTS=activity_cent USE_INTERCEPT=TRUE
  /RANDOM EFFECTS=activity_cent USE_INTERCEPT=TRUE
SUBJECTS=neigbourhood
    COVARIANCE_TYPE=UNSTRUCTURED
  /BUILD_OPTIONS TARGET_CATEGORY_ORDER=DESCENDING
INPUTS_CATEGORY_ORDER=ASCENDING
    MAX_ITERATIONS=100 CONFIDENCE_LEVEL=95 DF_METHOD=RESIDUAL
COVB=MODEL PCONVERGE=0.000001(ABSOLUTE)
    SCORING=0 SINGULAR=0.000000000001
  /EMMEANS_OPTIONS SCALE=ORIGINAL PADJUST=LSD.
```

Model summary

Target		health_dich
Probability distribution		Binomial
Link function		Logit
Information criterion	Akaike corrected	3065.897
	Bayesian	3079.437

Information criteria are based on the −2 log likelihood (3059.862) and are used to compare models. Models with smaller information criterion values fit better.

Fixed coefficients[a]

Model term	Coefficient	Std. error	t	Sig.	95% confidence interval	
					Lower	Upper
Intercept	0.191	0.1355	1.413	0.158	−0.075	0.458
activity_cent	0.163	0.0182	8.921	0.000	0.127	0.198

Probability distribution: binomial

Link function: Logit

[a] Target: health_dich

Random effect

Random effect covariance	Estimate	Std. error	Z	Sig.	95% confidence interval	
					Lower	Upper
UN (1,1)	0.466	0.207	2.247	0.025	0.195	1.115
UN (2,1)	−0.015	0.017	−0.862	0.389	−0.049	0.019
UN (2,2)	0.001	0.003	0.278	0.781	7.795E−7	1.049

Covariance structure: unknown

Subject specification: neigbourhood

Output 13.37 Syntax and result of a logistic mixed model analysis of the relationship between physical activity and the dichotomous health indicator with a random intercept and a random slope for activity on neighbourhood level performed with R

```
> out <- glmer(health_dich ~ activity_cent + (activity_cent|neighbourhood),
data=dataset, family=binomial, nAGQ=0)
```

```
Generalized linear mixed model fit by maximum likelihood (Adaptive Gauss-
Hermite Quadrature, nAGQ = 0) ['glmerMod']
 Family: binomial  ( logit )
Formula: health_dich ~ activity_cent + (activity_cent | neighbourhood)
   Data: dataset

    AIC      BIC   logLik deviance df.resid
   827.5    850.2   -408.8   817.5      679

Scaled residuals:
    Min      1Q  Median      3Q     Max
-2.9104 -0.8069  0.3932  0.7331  3.2584

Random effects:
 Groups        Name        Variance  Std.Dev. Corr
 neighbourhood (Intercept)  0.4997791 0.70695
               activity_cent 0.0005611 0.02369  -1.00
Number of obs: 684, groups:  neighbourhood, 48

Fixed effects:
              Estimate Std. Error z value Pr(>|z|)
(Intercept)    0.19208    0.13820   1.390    0.165
activity_cent  0.16309    0.01802   9.049   <2e-16 ***
---
Signif. codes:  0 '***' 0.001 '**' 0.01 '*' 0.05 '.' 0.1 ' ' 1

Correlation of Fixed Effects:
             (Intr)
activty_cnt -0.159
```

Table 13.10 Overview of the results of a logistic mixed model analysis of the relationship between physical activity (centred) and health, with a random intercept and random slope for activity on neighbourhood level estimated with different software packages

	Regression coefficient (SE)	Random variance		
		Intercept	Activity	Covariance
STATA	0.1714 (0.0207)	0.519	0.001	−0.018
SPSS	0.1630 (0.0182)	0.466	0.001	−0.015
R	0.1631 (0.0180)	0.500	0.001	−1.00*
SAS	0.1709 (0.0206)	0.502	0.001	−0.017

* R provides the correlation between random intercept and random slope instead of covariance.

Output 13.38 Syntax and result of a logistic mixed model analysis of the relationship between physical activity and the dichotomous health indicator with a random intercept on neighbourhood level performed with SAS

```
PROC GLIMMIX data = dich method=LAPLACE;
class neighbourhood;
model health_dich = activity_cent/s dist=binomial;
random int  activity_cent/ subject=neighbourhood type=un;
RUN;
```

Fit Statistics	
-2 Log Likelihood	817.37
AIC (smaller is better)	827.37
AICC (smaller is better)	827.46
BIC (smaller is better)	836.72
CAIC (smaller is better)	841.72
HQIC (smaller is better)	830.90

Solutions for Fixed Effects					
Effect	Estimate	Standard Error	DF	t Value	Pr > |t|
Intercept	0.1893	0.1423	47	1.33	0.1897
activity_cent	0.1709	0.02056	47	8.31	<.0001

Covariance Parameter Estimates			
Cov Parm	Subject	Estimate	Standard Error
UN(1,1)	neighbourhood	0.5020	0.2269
UN(2,1)	neighbourhood	-0.01662	0.01887
UN(2,2)	neighbourhood	0.000825	0.003406

Furthermore, in Chapter 5 it was shown that the effect estimates of a logistic mixed model analysis are an overestimation of the real effect estimates. So, in general, it is advised that the results of logistic mixed model analyses should be interpreted with great caution irrespective of the software program used.

References

Ahmed, I., Sutton, A. J. and Riley, R. (2011). Assessment of publication bias, selection bias, and unavailable data in meta-analyses using individual participant data: a database survey. *BMJ*, **344**, d7762.

Allison, P. D. (2001). *Missing Data*. Thousand Oaks, CA: Sage.

Atkinson, A. C. (1986). Masking unmasked. *Biometrika*, **73**, 533–541.

Audigier, V., White, I. R., Jolani, S., et al. (2017). Multiple imputation for multilevel data with continuous and binary variables. https://arxiv.org/abs/1702.00971

Barnett, V. and Lewis, T. (1994). *Outliers in Statistical Data*. New York: Wiley.

Browne, W. J. and Draper, D. (2006). A comparison of Bayesian and likelihood-based methods for fitting multilevel models. *Bayesian Analysis*, **3**, 473–514.

Bryk, A. S. and Raudenbush, S. W. (1992). *Hierarchical Linear Models*. Newbury Park, CA: Sage.

Burke, D. L., Ensor, J. and Riley, R. D. (2017). Meta-analysis using individual participant data: one-stage and two-stage approaches, and why they may differ. *Statistics in Medicine*, **36**, 855–875.

Cleves, M. A., Gould, W. W., Gutierrez, R. G. and Marchenko, Y. V. (2010). *An Introduction to Survival Analysis Using Stata*, 3rd edn. College Station, TX: Stata Press.

Cornell, J. E., Mulrow, C. D., Localio, R., et al. (2014). Random-effects meta-analysis of inconsistent effects: a time for change. *Annals of Internal Medicine*, **160**, 267–270.

Crouchley, R. and Davies, R. B. (2001). A comparison of GEE and random coefficient models for distinguishing heterogeneity, nonstationarity and state dependence in a collection of short binary event series. *Statistical Modelling*, **1**, 271–285.

Curran, P. J. and Bauer, D. J. (2001). The disaggregation of within-Person and between-Person effects in longitudinal models of change. *Annual Review of Psychology*, **62**, 583–619.

Debray, T. P. A., Moons, K. G. M., van Valkenhoef, G., et al. and the GetReal Methods Review Group (2015). Get real in individual participant data (IPD) meta-analysis: a review of the methodology. *Research Synthesis Methods*, **6**, 293–309.

Demidenko, E. (2013). *Mixed Models: Theory and Applications with R*, 2nd edn. Hoboken, NJ: Wiley.

Diez Roux, A. V. (2002). A glossary for multilevel analysis. *Journal of Epidemiology and Community Health*, **56**, 588–594.

Donders, A., van der Heiden, G., Stijnen, T. and Moons, K. (2012). Review: a gentle introduction to imputation of missing values. *Journal of Clinical Epidemiology*, **59**, 1087–1091.

Duncan, T., Duncan, S., Stryker, L., Li, F. and Alpert, A. (Eds.). (1999). *An Introduction to Latent Variable Modelling: Concepts, Issues and Applications*. Mahwah, NJ: Lawrence Erlbaum Associates.

Engel, B. (1998). A simple illustration of the failure of PQL, IRREML and AHPL as approximate ML methods for mixed models for binary data. *Biometrical Journal*, **40**, 141–154.

Fisher, D. J., Copas, A. J., Tierney, J. F. and Parmar, M. K. B. (2011). A critical review of methods for the assessment of patient-level interactions in individual participant data meta-analysis of randomized trials, and guidance for practitioners. *Journal of Clinical Epidemiology*, **64**, 949–967.

Galecki, A. and Burzykowski, T. (2013). *Linear Mixed-Effects Models Using R: A Step-by-Step Approach*. New York: Springer Texts in Statistics.

Gardner, W., Mulvey, E. P. and Shaw, E. C. (1995). Regression analyses of counts and rates: Poisson, overdispersed Poisson and negative binomial models. *Psychological Bulletin*, **118**, 392–404.

Gelwin, A. (2006). Prior distribution for variance parameters in hierarchical models (comment on article by Browne and Draper). *Bayesian Analysis*, **3**, 513–534.

Ghith, N., Wagner, P., Frølich, A. and Merlo, J. (2016). Short term survival after admission for heart failure in Sweden: applying multilevel analyses of discriminatory accuracy to evaluate institutional performance. *PLoS One*, **11**(2), e0148187.

Goldstein, H. (1987). *Multilevel Models in Educational and Social Research*. London/New York: Griffin/Oxford University Press.

Goldstein, H. (1992). Statistical information and the measurement of education outcomes (editorial). *Journal of the Royal Statistical Society, A*, **155**, 313–315.

Goldstein, H. (1995). *Multilevel Statistical Models*. London: Edward Arnold.

Goldstein, H. (2003). *Multilevel Statistical Models*, 3rd edn. London: Edward Arnold.

Goldstein, H. and Cuttance, P. (1988). A note on national assessment and school comparisons. *Journal of Education Policy*, **3**, 197–202.

Goldstein, H. and Rasbash, J. (1996). Improved approximation for multilevel models with binary responses. *Journal of the Royal Statistical Society, Series A*, **159**, 505–513.

Greenland, S. (2000a). When should epidemiologic regressions use random coefficients? *Biometrics*, **56**, 915–921.

Greenland, S. (2000b). Principles of multilevel modelling. *International Journal of Epidemiology*, **29**, 158–167.

Hedeker, D., Gibbons, R. D. and Waternaux, C. (1999). Sample size estimation for longitudinal designs with attrition: comparing time-related contrasts between groups. *Journal of Education and Behavioral Statistics*, **24**, 70–93.

Heo, M. and Leon, A. C. (2005). Comparison of statistical methods for analysis of clustered binary outcomes. *Statistics in Medicine*, **24**, 911–923.

Higgins, J. P. T., Whitehead, A., Turner, R. M., Omar, R. Z. and Thompson, S. G. (2001). Meta-analysis of continuous outcome data from individual patients. *Statistics in Medicine*, **20**, 2219–2241.

Hox, J. J. (2002). *Multilevel Analysis: Techniques and Applications*. Mahwah, NJ: Lawrence Erlbaum Associates.

Hu, F. B., Goldberg, J., Hedeker, D., Flay, B. R. and Pentz, M. A. (1998). Comparison of population-averaged and subject specific approaches for analyzing repeated measures binary outcomes. *American Journal of Epidemiology*, **147**, 694–703.

Hutchinson, M. K. and Holtman, M. C. (2005). Analysis of count data using poisson regression. *Research in Nursing & Health*, **28**, 408–418.

Jiang, J. (2007). *Linear and Generalized Linear Mixed Models and Their Applications*. New York: Springer-Verlag.

Jiang, J. (2016). *Robust Mixed Model Analysis*. World Scientific Publishing Co.

Jolani, S., Debray, T. P. A., Koffijberg, H., van Buuren, S. and Moons, K. G. M. (2015). Imputation of systematically missing predictors in an individual participant data meta-analysis: a generalized approach using MICE. *Statistics in Medicine*, **34**, 1841–1863.

Jöreskog, K. G. and Sörbom, D. (2001). *LISREL 8.5*. Chicago, IL: Scientific Software International.

Jung, S. H., Kang, S. H. and Ahn, C. (2001). Sample size calculations for clustered binary data. *Statistics in Medicine*, **20**, 1971–1982.

Kenward, M. G. and Roger, J. H. (1997). Small sample inference for fixed effects from restricted maximum likelihood. *Biometrics*, **53**, 983–997.

Korff, von, M., Koepsell, T., Curry, S. and Diehr, P. (1992). Multilevel analysis in epidemiologic research on health behaviors and outcomes. *American Journal of Epidemiology*, **135**, 1077–1082.

Kreft, I. and De Leeuw, J. (1998). *Introducing Multilevel Modelling*. London: Sage.

Lambert, P. C. and Royston, P. (2009). Further development of flexible parametric models for survival analysis. *Stata Journal*, **9**, 265–290.

Langford, I. H. and Lewis, T. (1998). Outliers in multilevel models (with discussion). *Journal of the Royal Statistical Society, A*, **161**, 121–160.

Larsen, K., Petersen, J. H., Budtz-Jorgensen, E. and Endahl, L. (2000). Interpreting parameters in the logistic regression model with random effects. *Biometrics*, **56**, 909–914.

Lawrence, A. J. (1995). Deletion, influence and masking in regression. *Journal of the Royal Statistical Society, B*, **57**, 181–189.

Lee, E. W. and Durbin, N. (1994). Estimation and sample size considerations for clustered binary responses. *Statistics in Medicine*, **13**, 1241–1252.

Lesaffre, E. and Spiessens, B. (2001). On the effect of the number of quadrature points in a logistic random-effects model: an example. *Applied Statistics*, **50**, 325–335.

Leyland, A. H. and Groenewegen, P. P. (2003). Multilevel modelling and public health policy. *Scandinavian Journal of Public Health*, **31**, 267–274.

Liang, K.-Y. and Zeger, S. L. (1993). Regression analysis for correlated data. *Annual Review of Public Health*, **14**, 43–68.

Lin, X. (1997). Variance component testing in generalised linear models with random effects. *Biometrika*, **84**, 309–325.

Lipsitz, S. R., Laird, N. M. and Harrington, D. P. (1991). Generalized estimating equations for correlated binary data: using the odds ratio as a measure of association. *Biometrika*, **78**, 153–160.

Littel, R. C., Pendergast, J. and Natarajan, R. (2000). Modelling covariance structures in the analysis of repeated measures data. *Statistics in Medicine*, **19**, 1793–1819.

Little, R. J. A. (1995). Modelling the drop-out mechanism repeated measures studies. *Journal of the American Statistical Association*, **90**, 1112–1121.

Little, R. J. A. and Rubin, D. B. (1987). *Statistical Analysis with Missing Data*. New York: Wiley.

Little, T. D., Schabel, K. U. and Baumert, J. (Eds.). (2000). *Modeling Longitudinal and Multilevel Data. Practical Issues, Applied Approaches, and Specific Examples*. Mahwah, NJ: Lawrence Erlbaum Associates.

Liu, G. and Liang, K.-Y. (1997). Sample size calculations for studies with correlated observations. *Biometrics*, **53**, 937–947.

Liu, Q. and Pierce, D. A. (1994). A note on Gauss-Hermite quadrature. *Biometrika*, **81**, 624–629.

Livert, D., Rindskopf, D., Saxe, L. and Stirratt, M. (2001). Using multilevel modelling in the evaluation of community-based treatment programs. *Multivariate Behavioral Research*, **36**, 155–183.

Ludtke, O., Marsh, H., Robitzsch, A., et al. (2008). The multilevel latent covariate model: a new, more reliable approach to group-level effects in contextual studies. *Psychological Methods*, **13**, 203–229.

McCullagh, P. and Searle, S. R. (2001). *Generalized, Linear and Mixed Models*. New York: Wiley.

Merlo, J. (2003). Multilevel analytical approaches in social epidemiology: measures of health variation compared with traditional measures of association. *Journal of Epidemiology and Community Health*, **57**, 550–552.

Moerbeek, M., Breukelen van, G. J. P. and Berger, M. P. F. (2000). Design issues for multilevel experiments. *Journal of Educational and Behavioral Statistics*, **25**, 271–284.

Moerbeek, M., Breukelen van, G. J. P. and Berger, M. P. F. (2001). Optimal experimental designs for multilevel logistic models. *The Statistician*, **50**, 17–30.

Moerbeek, M., van Breukelen, G. J. P. and Berger, M. P .F. (2003a). A comparison of estimation methods for multilevel logistic models. *Computational Statistics*, **18**, 19–37.

Moerbeek, M., van Breukelen, G. J. P., Ausems, M. and Berger, M. P. F. (2003b). Optimal sample sizes in experimental designs with individuals nested within clusters. *Understanding Statistics*, **2**, 151–175.

Morrell, C. H. (1998). Likelihood ratio testing of variance components in the linear mixed-effects model using restricted maximum likelihood. *Biometrics*, **54**, 1560–1568.

Muthén, B. (1984). A general structural equation model with dichotomous, ordered categorical, and continuous latent variable indicators. *Psychometrika*, **49**, 115–132.

Nelder, J. A. and Lee, Y. (1992). Likelihood, Quasi-likelihood and Pseudolikelihood: some comparisons. *Journal of the Royal Statistical Society, B*, **54**, 273–284.

Neuhaus, J. M., Kalbfleisch, J. D. and Hauck, W. W. (1991). A comparison of cluster-specific and population-averaged approaches for analyzing correlated binary data. *International Statistical Reviews*, **59**, 25–36.

Neuhaus, J. M. and Lesparance, M. L. (1996). Estimation efficiency in a binary mixed-effects model setting. *Biometrika*, **83**, 441–446.

Nuttall, D. L., Goldstein, H., Prosser, R. and Rasbash, J. (1989). Differential school effectiveness. *International Journal of Educational Research*, **13**, 769–776.

Oehlert, G. W. (2012). A few words about REML. *Stat 5303*, 1–11.

Omar, R. Z., Wright, E. M., Turner, R. M. and Thompson, S. G. (1999). Analyzing repeated measurements data: a practical comparison of methods. *Statistics in Medicine*, **18**, 1587–1603.

Pinheiro, J. C. and Bates, D. M. (2000). *Mixed-Effects Models in S and S-PLUS*. New York: Springer-Verlag.

Plewis, I. (1991). Using multilevel models to link educational progress with curriculum coverage. In *Schools, Classrooms and Pupils. International Studies of Schooling from a Multilevel Perspective*, ed. S. W. Raudenbush and J. D. Willms, San Diego: Academic Press.

Plewis, I. and Hurry, J. (1998). A multilevel perspective on the design and analysis of intervention studies. *Educational Research and Evaluation*, **4**, 13–26.

Rabe-Hesketh, S. and Pickles, A. (1999). Generalised linear latent and mixed models. In *Proceedings of the 14th International Workshop on Statistical Modelling*, ed. H. Friedl, A. Bughold and G. Kauermann, pp. 332–339. Graz, Austria: TU Graz Press.

Rabe-Hesketh, S., Pickles, A. and Taylor, C. (2000). sg129: generalized linear latent and mixed models. *Stata Technical Bulletin*, **53**, 47–57.

Rabe-Hesketh, S., Pickles, A. and Skrondal, A. (2001a). *GLAMM Manual Technical Report 2001/01*. Department of Biostatistics and Computing, Institute of Psychiatry, King's College, University of London.

Rabe-Hesketh, S., Pickles, A. and Skrondal, A. (2001b). GLLAMM: a class of models and a Stata program. *Multilevel Modelling Newsletter*, **13**, 17–23.

Rabe-Hesketh, S., Skrondal, A. and Pickles, A. (2002). Reliable estimation of generalized linear mixed models using adaptive quadrature. *The Stata Journal*, **2**, 1–21.

Rabe-Hesketh, S., Skrondal, A. and Pickles, A. (2004). *GLLAMM Manual*. U.C. Berekely Division of Biostatistics Working Paper Series, paper 160, www.bepres.com/ucbbiostat/paper160.

Rabe-Hesketh, S., Skrondal, A. and Pickles, A. (2005). Maximum likelihood estimation of limited and discrete dependent variable models with nested random effects. *Journal of Econometrics*, **128**, 301–323.

Raudenbush, S. W. and Bryk, A. S. (2002). *Hierarchical Linear Models. Applications and Data Analysis Methods*. Thousand Oaks, CA: Sage.

Reise, S. P. and Duan, N. (2003). *Multilevel Modelling Methodological Advances, Issues, and Applications*. Mahwah, NJ: Lawrence Erlbaum Associates.

Rice, N. and Leyland, A. (1996). Multilevel models: applications to health data. *Journal of Health Services Research Policy*, **1**, 154–164.

Riley, R. D., Lambert, P. C. and Abo-Zaid, G. (2010). Meta-analysis of individual participant data: rationale, conduct, and reporting. *BMJ*, **340**, c221.

Rodriguez, G. and Goldman, N. (1995). An assessment of estimation procedures for multilevel models with binary responses. *Journal of the Royal Statistical Association*, **158**, 73–89.

Rodriguez, G. and Goldman, N. (1997). Multilevel models with binary response: a comparison of estimation procedures. *Journal of the Royal Statistical Society, A*, **158**, 73–89.

Rodriguez, G. and Goldman, N. (2001). Improved estimation procedures for multilevel models with binary responses: a case study. *Journal of the Royal Statistical Association*, **164**, 339–355.

Royston, P. and Lambert, P. C. (2011). *Flexible Parametric Survival Analysis Using Stata: Beyond the Cox Model*. College Station, TX: Stata Press.

Rubin, D. B. (1987). *Multiple Imputation for Nonresponse in Surveys*. New York: Wiley.

Rubin, D. B. (1996). Multiple imputation after 18+ years. *Journal of the American Statistical Association*, **91**, 473–489.

Schafer, J. L. (1997). *Analysis of Incomplete Multivariate Data*. New York: Chapman & Hall.

Schafer, J. L. (1999). Multiple imputation: a primer. *Statistical Methods in Medical Research*, **8**, 3–15.

Schüle, S. A., von Kries, R., Fromme, H. and Bolte, G. (2016). Neighbourhood socioeconomic context, individual socioeconomic position, and overweight in young children: a multilevel study in a large German city. *BMC Obesity*, **3**, 25.

Shih, W. J. and Quan, H. (1997). Testing for treatment differences with dropouts present in clinical trials – a composite approach. *Statistics in Medicine*, **16**, 1225–1239.

Simmonds, M. C., Higgins, J. P. T., Stewart, L. A., et al. (2005). Meta-analysis of individual patient data from randomized trials: a review of methods used in practice. *Clinical Trials*, **2**, 209–217.

Simmonds, M., Stewart, G. and Stewart, L. (2015). A decade of individual participant data meta-analyses: a review of current practice. *Contemporary Clinical Trials*, **45**, 76–83.

Skrondal, A. and Rabe-Hesketh, S. (2004). *Generalized Latent Variable Modeling: Multilevel, Longitudinal and Structural Equation Models*. Boca Raton, FL: Chapman & Hall/CRC Press.

Snijders, T. A. B. and Bosker, R. J. (1993). Standard errors and sample sizes for two-level research. *Journal of Educational Statistics*, **18**, 237–259.

Snijders, T. A. B. and Bosker, R. J. (1999). *Multilevel Analysis. An Introduction to Basic and Advanced Multilevel Modelling*. London: Sage.

Sterne, J. A. C., White, I. A., Carlin, J. B., et al. (2009). Multiple imputation for missing data in epidemiological and clinical research: potential and pitfalls. *BMJ*, **338**, b2393.

Stewart, L. A. and Parmar, M. K. B. (1993). Meta-analysis of the literature or of individual patient data: is there a difference? *Lancet*, **341**, 418–422.

Steyerberg, E. W. (2009). *Clinical Prediction Models: A Practical Approach to Development, Validation, and Updating*. New York: Springer-Verlag.

Ten Have, T. R., Ratcliffe, S. J., Reboussin, B. A. and Miller, M. E. (2004). Deviations from the population-averaged cluster-specific relationship for clustered binary data. *Statistical Methods in Medical Research*, **13**, 3–16.

Twisk, J. W. R. (2004). Longitudinal data analysis. A comparison between generalized estimating equations and random coefficient analysis. *European Journal of Epidemiology*, **19**, 769–776.

Twisk, J. W. R. (2013). *Applied Longitudinal Data Analysis for Epidemiology: A Practical Guide*, 2nd edn. Cambridge: Cambridge University Press.

Twisk, J., de Boer, M., de Vente, W. and Heymans, M. (2013). Multiple imputation of missing values was not necessary before performing a longitudinal mixed-model analysis. *Journal of Clinical Epidemiology*, **66**, 1022–1028.

Twisk, J. W. R. and Proper, K. (2004). Evaluation of the results of a randomized controlled trial: how to define changes between baseline and follow-up. *Journal of Clinical Epidemiology*, **57**, 223–228.

Twisk, J. W. R. and de Vente, W. (2002). Attrition in longitudinal studies: how to deal with missing data. *Journal of Clinical Epidemiology*, **55**, 329–337.

Twisk, J. W. R., de Vente, W., Apeldoorn, A. T. and Boer, M. R. de (2017). Should we use logistic mixed model analysis for the effect estimation in a longitudinal RCT with a dichotomous outcome variable. *Epidemiology, Biostatistics and Public Health*, **14**, 3.

Weaver, C. G., Ravani, P., Oliver, M. J., Austin, P. C. and Quinn, R. R. (2015). Analyzing hospitalisation data: potential limitations of Poisson regression. *Nephrology Dialysis Transplantation*, **30**, 1244–1249.

West, B. T., Welch, K. B. and Galecki, A. T. (2015). *Linear Mixed Models: A Practical Guide Using Statistical Software*, 2nd edn. Boca Raton, FL: CRC Press.

Woodhouse, G. and Goldstein, H. (1989). Educational Performance Indicators and LEA league tables. *Oxford Review of Education*, **14**, 301–319.

Zeger, S. L. and Liang, K.-Y. (1986). Longitudinal data analysis for discrete and continuous outcomes. *Biometrics*, **42**, 121–130.

Zeger, S. L. and Liang, K.-Y. (1992). An overview of methods for the analysis of longitudinal data. *Statistics in Medicine*, **11**, 1825–1839.

Zheng, X. and Rabe-Hesketh, S. (2007). Estimating parameters of dichotomous and ordinal item response models with gllamm. *The Stata Journal*, **3**, 313–333.

Index